MW00778682

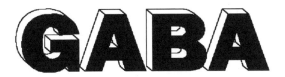

The
ANXIETY
Amino Acid

by

Billie Jay Sahley, Ph.D.
with
Katherine M. Birkner, C.R.N.A., Ph.D.

Pain & Stress Publications®
San Antonio, Texas
2001

Note to Readers

This material is not intended to replace the services of a physician, nor is it meant to encourage diagnosis and treatment of illness, disease, or other medical problems by the layman. This book should not be regarded as a substitute for professional medical treatment. While every care is taken to ensure the accuracy of the content, the author and the publishers cannot accept legal responsibility for any problem arising out of experimentation with the methods described. Any application of the recommendations set forth in the following pages is at the reader's discretion and sole risk. If you are under a physician's care for any condition, he or she must advise you whether the program described in this book is suitable for you or your child. If you are taking prescription medications, DO NOT STOP THE MEDICATION without a physician's assistance.

This publication has been compiled through research resources at the Pain & Stress Center, San Antonio, Texas.

The names of the patients described in this book have been changed to protect their privacy.

First Edition, January 1998
Second Edition, June 2001

Additional copies may be ordered from:
Pain & Stress Center
5282 Medical Drive, Suite 160, San Antonio, Texas 78229-6023
1-800-669-2256 or
http://www.painstresscenter.com

Library of Congress Catalog Card Number 2001117704

ISBN 1-889391-17-4

Contents

Dedication

I have been very blessed over the past twenty years to have associates, staff, and friends that are dedicated to finding natural alternatives to help those who suffer.

I would like to express special thanks to the people who helped make this book possible:

> To Katherine M. Birkner, C.R.N.A., Ph.D. who has been an angel on my shoulder spending countless hours helping me do research, and constantly encouraging me to continue conquering my impossible dream.

> To my staff who has given many unselfish hours reading, proofing, and making helpful suggestions.

> To my friends and fellow health care practitioners who have constantly encouraged me to continue research with GABA and other amino acids to replace drugs.

> To all of these gifted and special people.

> And to the Lord for always lighting my path, I dedicate this book.

Introduction

The last 20 years of my life encompassed a chain of events that inspired me to begin a search for answers to chronic stress, anxiety, and brain function.

I suppose I have always been interested in emotions and behavior. Even as a child of twelve, after major surgery on my neck, I remember asking my mother, "What makes people do and feel what they do?" All through high school, I knew I wanted to study behavior and brain function, and upon entering college, I proceeded to do so.

Then, in the seventies I faced multiple personal crises that caused me to experience irrational behavior. I lost my mother after her five-year battle with cancer. She was all I had left after I lost my father when I was six. My stepfather decided to make my life hell on earth, which he did, and that ended any and all contact with him. While driving on the expressway, I was hit by a gravel truck and went through the windshield. I lay there for an hour before they could get me out. At first, they didn't rush because they thought I was dead. When they realized I was still alive, they tried to go too fast, thus causing more injuries.

Needless to say, my neck and back have never been the same. I could not understand or correct the mental stress and physical symptoms that caused my irrational behavior. Time after time doctors offered prescription drugs for pain, depression, grief, and my constant companion—anxiety. My answer was the same—NO, that's not the answer.

I knew I had to resolve these behaviors and let it go so I could heal and live in peace. I knew drugs would only cause me to repress and suppress the pain of the past, and the pain would still be very much alive in my subconscious. To be whole again, I had to put closure on those ten years of hell.

My search for answers to my subconscious overload intensified. How were my thoughts and feelings influencing my immune system? What could I feed my brain to restore homeostasis?

Then I was introduced to psychopharmacology, a field of research that uses drugs and other chemical agents that enable researchers to investigate how the brain functions. I focused on other chemical agents and experienced my first real addiction—*research,* and the possibility of charting results of biochemicals that not only alter behavior, but also influence the immune system. I found my missing link—the study of mind-body medicine. At the same time the field of psychoneuroimmunology was becoming a specialty, and researchers from behavioral medicine, immunology, and neurology were working together to explore the mind-body connection. Then the field of orthomolecular therapy exploded. I spent every spare minute I had doing research with amino acids and how they can and do affect mind, mood, memory, and behavior. I attended every conference I could and talked with researchers all over the country about the brain and nutrient connection.

As time passed, the pieces began to fall into place and presented a clear picture of brain function. Researchers found and proved that neurotransmitters and neuropeptides were the key to behavior, emotions, and pain. Freedom from prescription drugs for anxiety became a reality, and a new breed of health practitioners arrived.

My plans for the future include focusing my time and energy on research, product development, and writing. The rewards for this are the thousands of patients who have been and will be helped, and who live and will live drug-free.

You encounter many people on a journey such as mine—all of them offer valuable insight. But then, I had the opportunity to meet someone who had a major impact on my life, and takes you to another level. I was blessed with meeting and working with gifted healers—Julian Whitaker, M.D., Candace Pert, Ph.D., Doris Rapp, M.D., Sherry Rogers, M.D., and Jeffrey S. Bland, Ph.D.

Dr. Whitaker has a true gift of healing, and has helped millions of people, using only nutritional supplements. His constant encouragement helped me to continue my extensive research and product development to help those who suffer. Dr. Candace Pert is a brilliant neuroscientist and a pioneer in how thoughts and emotions affect our health. Dr. Pert's dedication to her research allowed her to find the GABA receptor sites, as well as many other important receptors. I have followed her work for years, and she has always inspired me. One of the most exciting events in my life was meeting Dr. Pert at an Environmental Medicine meeting, and sharing ideas with her. I gave Dr. Pert a bottle of Anxiety Control. She looked at the formula and said, "You're right on track." After her comment, I didn't need a plane to fly home! Dr. Pert's revolutionary research establishes the crucial link between the mind and body, and how our feelings can affect our health. I think she deserves a Nobel Prize for all of her research and the wealth of information she has shared relating to the crucial link between mind and body.

Dr. Sherry Rogers introduced me to the importance of magnesium for anxiety as well as many other important functions in the body. Over the years Dr. Rogers research has been a great help to my own work in brain research. Dr. Rogers has a special gift for finding vital research and sharing it.

Dr. Doris Rapp introduced me to the work of environmental medicine including environmental chemicals, allergies, especially food allergies. Dr. Rapp's work with children furthered my knowledge about allergies and how they affect the brain and behavior.

Dr. Jeffrey Bland opened the door to the field of advanced nutritional biochemistry and functional medicine.

Over the past twenty years I have found research regarding brain function and development to be one of the most rewarding experiences of my professional life. As a scientist I look forward each day to the new discoveries—especially my new developments that explain human behavior, health, and wellness. As we move into the new century, the doors to natural alternatives for stress, anxiety, fear, and depression continue to open and those who suffer will find the natural solutions they need to heal *drug-free*.

The Brain and Limbic System Pathways

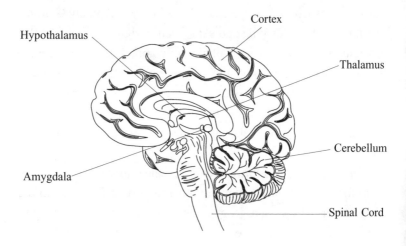

Brain function depends on brain nutrition.
There is no such thing as a tranquilizer or Xanax deficiency!

1
What are Amino Acids?

Amino Acids are the building blocks of protein and are essential to life. Proteins regulate every action that occurs in the body. Amino acids make up 75% of what remains in the body after you remove the fat and water. Proteins are found in the skeletal muscles and the structural tissues of the body. Body functions supported by amino acids depend on proper amino acid metabolism.

Essential amino acids must be obtained from your diet or in supplement form. Metabolic impairments are hidden in many individuals, and may be subtle, or they can surface as an overt disease. An amino acid analysis should be considered if there is a possibility of dysfunctional amino acid metabolism including chronic fatigue, headaches, chronic gastrointestinal distress, food

Classification of Amino Acids

NonEssential	Conditionally Essential	Essential
Alanine	Arginine	Histidine
Asparagine	Cysteine	Isoleucine
Aspartic Acid	Cystine	Leucine
Glutamic Acid	GABA	Lysine
Glycine	Glutamine	Methionine
Proline	Taurine	Phenylalanine
Serine	Tyrosine	Threonine
		Tryptophan
		Valine

allergies, inflammatory responses, depression, learning disabilities, protein malabsorption, neurological disorders, or symptoms of degenerative disease. Essential amino acids cannot be formed in the body and must be obtained from the diet. If you have low levels of essential and conditionally essential amino acids, this indicates improper ingestion.

Disorders Associated with Amino Acid Deficiencies

- ADD/ADHD
- Alcoholism
- Ammonia toxicity
- Anxiety, fear, and panic
- Ataxia (defective muscular coordination)
- Behavioral disorders
- Cardiovascular disease
- Chemical intolerances
- Chronic fatigue
- Chronic gastrointestinal distress or bowel irregularity
- Depression
- Dermatitis (inflammation of the skin)
- Detoxification impairments
- Excessive inflammation
- Failure to thrive (infancy)
- Family history or early symptoms of degenerative disease
- Frequent headaches
- Frequent infections and persistent inflammatory responses
- Hyperlipidemia (high blood lipid levels)
- Hypertension (high blood pressure)
- Hypotonia (loss of muscle tone)
- Inflammatory disorders
- Impaired mental development
- Insomnia
- Intolerances (persistent) to foods and chemicals
- Mental misperception
- Mental retardation
- Myopathies (muscular diseases)
- Neurological disorders
- Neural tube defects (birth defects)
- Ocular disorders (eye)
- Osteoporosis
- Oxidative stress
- Poor immunity
- Poor wound healing
- Rheumatoid arthritis
- Seizures
- Short stature or chronically underweight, growth failure (children)
- Weak skin and nails

Source: Great Smokies Diagnostic Laboratory

2
GABA Discovery

The first time I became aware of the amino acid, GABA, was in 1982 when one of my patients came in very excited and asked if I had seen the information regarding GABA for anxiety. He told me about a book that had just been released by Durk Pearson and Sandy Shaw, researchers in nutritional biochemistry at M.I.T.

The book, *Life Extension*, was well on its way to becoming a million plus seller. As soon as possible, I went to the bookstore and purchased a copy. There it was on page 755, a paragraph describing documented research on GABA for anxiety.

"Recently, researchers have found out about some of these natural substances which fit the benzodiazepine receptors. One is niacinamide. The vitamin, inositol, and the amino acid, GABA, enhance niacinamide binding to the benzodiazepine receptors. Niacinamide, inositol, and GABA can therefore, at least partly, replace Valium or Librium by binding the same receptors and providing tranquilization. Mr. P has tried this. He says that he is less depressed than before, no longer suffering from monthly deep depressions but only occasional shallow ones. His friends have commented on this improvement. He has been able to cut his alcohol use in half. Mr. P says that GABA feels very similar to Valium, but does not quite give him the energy that he gets from Valium. Finally, Mr. P uses C, B1, and cysteine at times when he is drinking and has found it makes it easier for him to get up in the morning (after a bad day) to go to his office."

From that day forward my life has never been the same. I began an intensive search for any and all information about GABA, anxiety, and how it relates to behavior. That search is ongoing, and I am sure it will continue for years to come. Not only has my research led me to use GABA for anxiety, but I've learned how important this inhibitory neurotransmitter is to those who suffer from depression, pain, panic, addiction, hyperactivity, and ADD. GABA makes a major difference in our stress and anxiety-filled world.

GABA and other inhibitory neurotransmitters such as glutamine, glycine, taurine, tryptophan, and tyrosine already replace many antidepressants and tranquilizers that are over-prescribed today. The American public is now aware of the positive results of natural alternatives to prescription drugs for chronic stress and anxiety. Over the past ten years, the numbers of people seeking alternative therapy practitioners has increased by 60%. People realize the importance of feeding the brain needed nutrients rather than just suppressing symptoms with prescribed addictive drugs.

According to the Anxiety Disorders Association of America, anxiety and panic disorders are the number one mental health problem in the United States. This pervasive problem affects at least nineteen million people ages 16 to 60 each year from all walks of life. Children are not immune to anxiety. The latest research reports demonstrate approximately 13 million youngsters ages 10 to 18 have anxiety-related problems. Numerous times teachers mistake anxiety behavior as ADD and ADHD. This problem continues to grow in children. Children who have not developed communication skills and are unable to express their feelings, especially fear-related anger and anxiety, are most at risk. Often, a genetic link from a parent or grandparent predisposes children to anxiety.

Brain Command Center

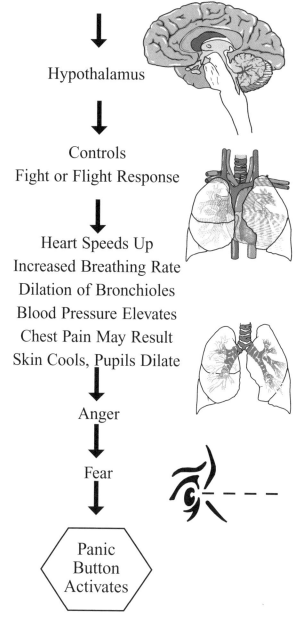

Low GABA levels decrease serotonin levels.

Low serotonin increases anger and feelings of loss of control.

Loss of control causes anxiety and fear that triggers panic or the fight-or-flight response.

Low GABA levels trigger increased epinephrine and norepinephrine release; that in turn, decreases logical thinking and increases heart rate.

Hypothalamus

↓

Controls
Fight or Flight Response

↓

Heart Speeds Up
Increased Breathing Rate
Dilation of Bronchioles
Blood Pressure Elevates
Chest Pain May Result
Skin Cools, Pupils Dilate

↓

Anger

↓

Fear

↓

Panic
Button
Activates

All of this occurs in a split second.

This being said parents must realize drugs like Ritalin and Adder-all are not the answers. *There is no such thing as a stimulant deficiency. The key is nourishing the brain with the nutrients it needs to make vital neurotransmitters.*

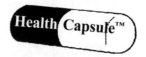

Anxiety is an equal opportunity offender,
exempting no one on the basis of
age, sex, race, or religion.

Acceptance of anxiety and fear is a
switch that shuts them off.

3
GABA

For more than a half century, scientists have known about GABA in plant form. In 1950 Eugene Roberts, Ph.D., a distinguished scientist at Washington University in St. Louis, discovered Gamma Amino Butyric Acid—GABA. In 1956 researchers demonstrated GABA was involved in the condition of nerve impulses. The next ten years of research provided scientists the information needed to establish GABA as a major inhibitory neurotransmitter that has widespread distribution throughout the brain and body.

In the early 1970s, Candace B. Pert, while a student in pharmacology at John Hopkins University, discovered GABA receptor sites throughout the brain and body. Dr. Pert's research continued to demonstrate the importance of GABA for multiple uses in the stress-anxiety network.

The study of GABA and other amino acids and how they affect the brain chemistry provides a focal project for many medical researchers. GABA (Gamma Amino Butyric Acid) is an inhibitory neurotransmitter, and is found throughout the central nervous system. Forty to fifty percent of all brain synapses contain GABA. GABA, the most widely distributed neurotransmitter in the brain, plays an important role in neuronal and behavioral inhibition. GABA is present in a concentration some 200 to 1000 times greater than neurotransmitters such as acetylcholine, noradrenaline, and 5-HTP. The highest concentrations of GABA reside in the basal ganglia followed by the hypothalamus, hippocampus, cortex, amygdala, and thalamus. GABA's highest concentration in the hypothalamus reflects the significant role in hypothalamic-pituitary function. The hypothalamus is the region of the brain that regulates instinctive functions such as sleep-wake cycles, body temperature, and the activity of the pituitary gland.

Feelings of fear, anxiety, anger, grief, depression, and elation all dwell in the storehouse of emotion—the amygdala. The amygdala is part of the limbic system, and it influences some of the most complex functions of the brain.

Dr. Pert's later research disclosed that the hippocampus in the limbic system provides the access or gateway into our emotional experiences. Emotional memories, traumatic episodes, or any experience that causes you to feel a loss of control, is recorded for playback in the limbic system network at a later date. Traumatic memories can be stored in many places, not just in the brain, but also in the stomach, skin, muscles, or any organ. Since GABA receptor sites reside throughout your brain and body, taking GABA in therapeutic amounts reduces the amount of stress and anxiety on any organ. GABA is the most common message-altering neurotransmitter in the brain.

Dr. Michael Gershon, a professor of anatomy and cell biology at Columbia Presbyterian Medical Center in New York, maintains the body has two brains, one in the skull, and one in the human gut. When one gets upset, so does the other. In his best-selling book, *The Second Brain,* Dr. Gershon reports many gastrointestinal disorders like colitis, irritable bowel syndrome, and diverticulitis, originate from problems within the gut's brain.

The gut's brain is located in sheaths of tissue lining the esophagus, stomach, small intestine, and the colon. GABA, other amino acids, and neurotransmitters flow freely in this complex network. A short supply of GABA and the needed neurotransmitters can upset the stress networks of both brains. The brain in the head communicates with the brain in the stomach through neurons and neurotransmitters that relay messages back and forth. An upset stomach or diarrhea can be the direct result of prolonged anxiety and overloaded circuits in the head brain. When using antidepressants or tranquilizers for various reasons, the stomach brain rejects these chemicals by sending signals of upset, heartburn, gas, or bloating. GABA has a calming effect on the stomach, and many people who have a nervous stomach use a little GABA prior to meals. The suggested dose is ¼ to ½ capsule of pure pharmaceutical grade GABA, depending on your body weight, *or* use 1 capsule of Anxiety Control. This relaxes the stomach muscles and replenishes this important neurotransmitter.

Both the head and stomach brains represent a network of your emotions, both expressed and repressed. Your behavior is a direct result of your stress levels, your unnourished brains, and unresolved anxiety. Repressed anger can cause an intestinal malfunction as well as symptoms of irritable bowel syndrome (IBS) or spastic colon. Feelings of hostility and anger that cannot be expressed attack the enteric nervous system further depleting GABA and other neurotransmitter stores. Chronic diarrhea and a feeling of butterflies in the stomach are part of the stress-anxiety cycle. Dr. Gershon's research into the second brain and the importance of amino acids, especially GABA and serotonin, provides an in depth understanding for those suffering from chronic anxiety and gut-related problems.

Why Amino Acid Deficiencies Occur—

- Inborn metabolic errors or genetic predisposition to amino acid deficiencies.

- Poor dietary habits—overconsumption of processed or junk foods, alcohol, and soft drinks.

- Inadequate digestion and absorption of proteins.

- Inadequate cofactors, B6 or P5'P, and magnesium.

- Chronic stress, anxiety, illness, hyperactivity, or disease.

Anatomy of Anxiety and Brain Function

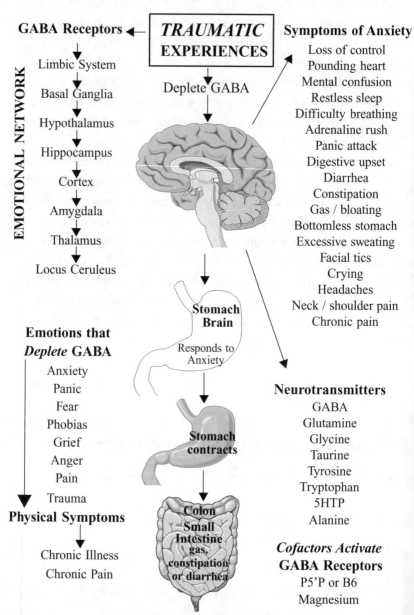

GABA Receptors ← **TRAUMATIC EXPERIENCES**

EMOTIONAL NETWORK

Limbic System
↓
Basal Ganglia
↓
Hypothalamus
↓
Hippocampus
↓
Cortex
↓
Amygdala
↓
Thalamus
↓
Locus Ceruleus

Deplete GABA

Symptoms of Anxiety

Loss of control
Pounding heart
Mental confusion
Restless sleep
Difficulty breathing
Adrenaline rush
Panic attack
Digestive upset
Diarrhea
Constipation
Gas / bloating
Bottomless stomach
Excessive sweating
Facial tics
Crying
Headaches
Neck / shoulder pain
Chronic pain

Stomach Brain

Responds to Anxiety

Stomach contracts

Colon Small Intestine gas, constipation or diarrhea

Emotions that *Deplete* GABA

Anxiety
Panic
Fear
Phobias
Grief
Anger
Pain
Trauma

Physical Symptoms

Chronic Illness
Chronic Pain

Neurotransmitters

GABA
Glutamine
Glycine
Taurine
Tyrosine
Tryptophan
5HTP
Alanine

***Cofactors Activate* GABA Receptors**

P5'P or B6
Magnesium

Psychiatric drugs work by effecting GABA
and other amino acids and their receptors.

4
Major Inhibitory Neurotransmitter

GABA is the major inhibitory neurotransmitter that influences brain function. GABA performs biochemical and metabolic actions in the brain and body in addition to its neurotransmitter function. These particular characteristics of GABA have major implications for biological psychiatry. The brain contains fifty plus neurotransmitters and new ones are being discovered daily.

We characterize neurotransmitters as excitatory or inhibitory. GABA's major function regulates and inhibits anxiety, muscle spasm, fear, panic, depression, and alcohol addiction. Chronic stress syndrome and anxiety tremendously increase GABA requirements in the brain and body. We are all biochemically unique and no two people require the same amount of amino acids. Each individual's distinct chemical composition and brain functions prove unique to their lifestyle and nutrient intake. The effectiveness of brain function has a direct relationship to the number of neurons it has. Neurons come from neurotransmitters via amino acids. The brain cannot store vital neurotransmitters. Amino acids must be supplied on a daily basis through supplementation. Millions of times a second, signals fire within the brain, composing a complex symphony of messages involving mental, emotional, and physical events. Neurotransmitter synthesis occurs within the neuron from precursors delivered to the cell from the outside.

GABA is the major inhibitory neurotransmitter because of its inhibitory action on the limbic system, amygdala, locus ceruleus, and hippocampus. This action inhibits or slows down the constant firing of anxiety and panic-related messages at the cortex, the decision-making part of the brain. GABA fills the group of receptor sites in the brain that slows down and blocks excitatory messages trying to reach the limbic system. Therefore, when the cortex receives a message, it does not overwhelm you with anxiety, panic, pain, or craving. Since the stomach has a brain of its own and numerous receptor sites that require GABA, adequate amounts must be used on a regular basis. Our research at the Pain & Stress Center over the past ten years provided excellent results with anxiety prone patients. We use GABA, 375 and 750 mg. This pure pharmaceutical grade GABA is tasteless and dissolves readily in water, tea, or any liquid. Start with one 375 mg or half a capsule will give you relief in 10 to 12 minutes. *Be patient. Do not overdose or you will have side effects.* Anytime you use an amino acid such as GABA, you must use B6 or P5'P (Pyridoxal 5 Phosphate) for a cofactor; otherwise, your body cannot metabolize it properly. Magnesium, especially magnesium chloride, also enhances the effects of GABA. This combination is excellent for muscle spasms, nervous stomach as well as for anxiety attacks. Ninety-five percent of Pain & Stress Center patients followed for five years with acute symptoms of anxiety, also presented with symptoms of magnesium deficiency. This mineral and GABA are an excellent combination for the relief of stress, anxiety, grief, depression, and pain.

Julian Whitaker, M.D., in his newsletter, *Health and Healing,* March 1994, recommends GABA as an excellent resource for anxiety prone individuals. Dr. Whitaker describes the pitfalls of benzodiazepines that only mimic the actions and functions of GABA by attaching to the GABA receptor sites in the brain. Why use a drug that only attaches when you can fill the receptor site with what belongs there—GABA. The drug companies call the GABA receptor site, the benzodiazepine receptor site. There is no benzodiazepine receptor site. Benzodiazepines include Xanax, Ativan, Librium, Tranxene, Valium, Restoril, Paxipam, Dalmane, Halcion, and Klonopin.

Max Ricketts in his best selling book, *The Great Anxiety Escape,* outlines a nutritional support program to help those who suffer from anxiety and panic, as he once did. The program describes the effectiveness of GABA and other amino acids for anxiety. Max Ricketts' book emphasizes the biochemistry of the brain can be altered by nutrient intake, and how prolonged anxiety can cause an imbalance. Ricketts, who was once addicted to benzodiazepines for his anxiety and panic, describes his long journey through his addiction to total recovery using amino acids and nutrients, as well as other stress-releasing techniques. His message is clear—the roots of anxiety disorders lie in chemical imbalances within the brain and body.

The pervasive use of benzodiazepines and SSRIs for anxiety has reached an all time high in the United States. Last year more than 80 million prescriptions for benzodiazepines were filled. Xanax for anxiety was right at the top. The January 1993 *Consumer Reports* reported extensive studies that demonstrated the ineffectiveness of Xanax, Prozac, and Halcion, as well as many other drugs that were not effective. Drugs only block symptoms; they do not correct the imbalance. Stop the drugs and the symptoms return. Those who suffer from anxiety need neurotransmitters to restore their balance of the brain chemistry. Amino acids create needed neurotransmitters. Drugs do not; they *only use* the available neurotransmitters. Given all of research data available regarding the adverse side effects, as well as a possibility of addiction, should not your choice be to restore the brain chemistry to its natural state, rather than just suppress symptoms?

GABA is the most prevalent inhibitory neurotransmitter in the brain. According to Michael J. Gitlin, M.D., in *The Psychotherapist's Guide to Psychopharmacology*, GABA appears to "have a specific role to play in the regulation of anxiety. GABA inhibits activity at the locus ceruleus, the area thought to be centrally involved in panic attacks." Dr. Gitlin describes the locus ceruleus as part of the brain with the highest concentration of cells using norepinephrine as a neurotransmitter. When the locus ceruleus, the brain's alarm, is stimulated, fear responses such as elevated blood pressure, rapid breathing, and sweating result. Dr. Gitlin postulates mitral valve prolapse may be associated with panic disorder. Millions of women suffer from this problem and have intense anxiety from skipped heartbeats. Anxiety can and does provoke mitral valve prolapse. Many patients respond to GABA and magnesium to slow down the incoming signals, and reduce both the anxiety and the condition of mitral valve prolapse. Research demonstrates a magnesium deficiency is a common occurrence in people with mitral value prolapse, and in numerous cases is responsible for many of the symptoms. A correction with magnesium chloride plus a decrease in anxiety using the right GABA formula will improve the condition. The combination I find to be the most effective is Anxiety Control, Mag Link, and 5-HTP. 5-HTP is for serotonin enhancement.

Sitting at the base of the brain is a tiny bean-shaped pod that is part of the limbic network. The locus ceruleus goes into high gear when prolonged anxiety and stress deplete GABA stores. GABA not only effectively manages anxiety, but epilepsy, hypertension, and attention deficit disorder. For those with a decreased sex drive, GABA regulates the release of sex hormones. This information was reported in *Prescription for Nutritional Healing A to Z, Guide to Supplements,* by James Balch, M.D., and Phyllis Balch, C.N.C. Research done by Harold Whitcomb, M.D., and Phyllis Bronson, Ph.D., a nutritional biochemist at the Aspen Clinic for Preventive and Environmental Medicine, disclosed that women approaching menopause have estrogen levels that are too high and progesterone levels that are too low. This can predispose them to anxiety and panic. The anxiety can be generated by a deficiency of GABA and its inhibitory activity in the brain. A deficiency of GABA can

How Anxiety Effects the Nervous System and Organs

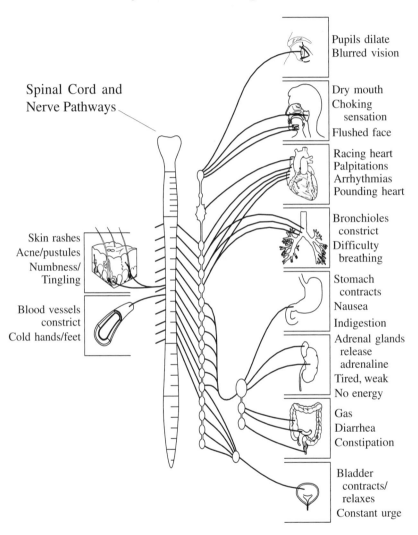

Spinal Cord and Nerve Pathways

Pupils dilate
Blurred vision

Dry mouth
Choking
  sensation
Flushed face

Racing heart
Palpitations
Arrhythmias
Pounding heart

Bronchioles
  constrict
Difficulty
  breathing

Skin rashes
Acne/pustules
Numbness/
  Tingling

Blood vessels
constrict
Cold hands/feet

Stomach
  contracts
Nausea
Indigestion

Adrenal glands
  release
  adrenaline
Tired, weak
No energy

Gas
Diarrhea
Constipation

Bladder
  contracts/
  relaxes
Constant urge

There are GABA receptors in each organ. Anxiety, panic, fear, anger, grief, pain, and depression effect all organs of the nervous system. Candace Pert states, "Emotions are the connection between the mind and the body, and there is no separation between the two. Mind doesn't dominant body, it *becomes* body—body and mind are one."

cause a person to feel the sensation that their brain is racing and out of control. GABA produces a calming effect on the brain by inhibiting the production of excitatory brain chemicals. These other chemicals tend to increase the brain's activities, causing a feeling of loss of control.

A large number of patients appear to suffer from deficiencies or abnormalities in their neurotransmitters—especially the vaso-constrictor serotonin produced by tryptophan, 5-HTP, as well as GABA. Recent research establishes the precise relationship between hormones, moods, and neurotransmitters. This research is at the cutting edge of brain research and anxiety behavior. Men have much less control over their emotions than women, and will aggressively act out anger and anxiety. Then men turn to alcohol and drugs for relief. Women demonstrate a variety of emotional ailments such as panic attacks, depression, and eating disorders. Women must contend with faulty estrogen and progesterone imbalances that influence their brain chemistry and behavior. Patients at the Pain & Stress Clinic over 40 years old showed a remarkable improvement after adding DHEA (Dehydroepiandrosterone). DHEA is the most abundant hormone in humans. GABA increases DHEA levels in the brain as well as the amino acids, tyrosine, arginine, ornithine, and lysine.

In an interview with *Alternative Medicine Digest,* Dr. Whitcomb described a typical patient at Aspen Clinic: a 42-year-old female who presented with a history of anxiety, panic attacks, and a very low progesterone level. The patient's medical history revealed her anxiety was exacerbated by a shortage of GABA. Further evaluation revealed the patient was estrogen dominant. Estrogen dominant women have unusually low levels of amino acids in the inhibitory class—GABA, glutamine, glycine, and taurine. The prolonged stress and anxiety of impending menopause can cause numerous nutrient imbalances such as magnesium, especially magnesium chloride. Dr. Whitcomb placed the patient on

GABA along with a combination formula and other nutrients. She had a marked improvement and a decrease in her anxiety, panic, and a racing heart.

At the Pain & Stress Center we see a large number of patients with similar symptoms. Our treatment protocol includes GABA, Anxiety Control, and Mag Link. We also add superhormones such as DHEA and Pregnenolone as part of the program, if needed. Both perimenopausal and menopausal women with a marked decline in hormones are receptive to superhormones such as DHEA and Pregnenolone. According to William Regelson, M.D., in his book, *The Super Hormone Promise,* "Superhormones are similar to neurotransmitters and have a profound impact on mental function. GABA cools the brain and protects our nerve cells from burning out in the course of all the activity. Pregnenolone mitigates the effects of GABA and restores balance to the brain chemistry."

Scientific researchers in the field of psychopharmacology continue to uncover important documentation regarding GABA as the master controller that oversees brain function. *U.S. News & World Report*, August 18, 1997, published a story entitled, "How Does Anesthesia Work?" by Mary Brophy Marcus. "All general anesthetics appear to shut off the brain from external stimuli. One way they do this is by altering the chemistry of the synapses, the gap between nerve cells. Chemicals called neurotransmitters normally act as messengers, crossing the synapse to relay a nerve signal. Other brain chemicals, in particular one called GABA, tend to shut off the signal. Many anesthetics appear to block the excitatory neurotransmitter or enhance the natural effects of GABA." The importance of GABA and brain function continues to grow as researchers uncover more of this amazing amino acid's major influence on the brain and body chemistry.

Actress Margot Kidder suffered from episodes of bipolar disorder, chronic stress, and hormonal imbalances prior to her periods. She tried conventional therapies and drugs, but never

Amino Acids for
Brain and Body Function

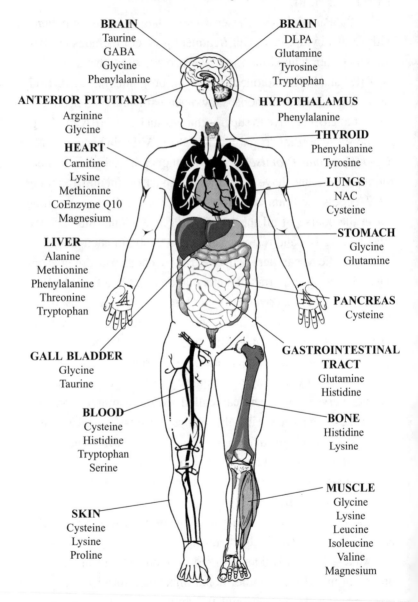

BRAIN
Taurine
GABA
Glycine
Phenylalanine

BRAIN
DLPA
Glutamine
Tyrosine
Tryptophan

ANTERIOR PITUITARY
Arginine
Glycine

HYPOTHALAMUS
Phenylalanine

THYROID
Phenylalanine
Tyrosine

HEART
Carnitine
Lysine
Methionine
CoEnzyme Q10
Magnesium

LUNGS
NAC
Cysteine

STOMACH
Glycine
Glutamine

LIVER
Alanine
Methionine
Phenylalanine
Threonine
Tryptophan

PANCREAS
Cysteine

GALL BLADDER
Glycine
Taurine

**GASTROINTESTINAL
TRACT**
Glutamine
Histidine

BLOOD
Cysteine
Histidine
Tryptophan
Serine

BONE
Histidine
Lysine

MUSCLE
Glycine
Lysine
Leucine
Isoleucine
Valine
Magnesium

SKIN
Cysteine
Lysine
Proline

Always add magnesium and B6 or P5'P to all amino acids.

improved. Her problems began as a teenager. Her physician started her on Valium, and told her it was not addictive. It took her more than 10 years to free herself from the Valium. After many years of multiple diagnoses and no improvement, she began to do research on her own. This led her to orthomolecular therapy.

Her research led her to GABA and its effect on the dopamine levels in the brain. Margot found when your GABA level is low in the brain; you will experience anxiety, nervousness, and agitation. She began taking GABA and taurine, both inhibitory neurotransmitters as well as B complex to restore her very deficient brain. After a year, she reduced her medications and felt much better. Her journey into the world of orthomolecular medicine led her to Dr. Abram Hoffer, one of the founders of Orthomolecular Medicine. Dr. Hoffer started Margot on a complete regimen to build up her nutritional status. Today, Margot is alive and well, and her healing is a very important aspect of her life. Her doctor confirmed she had extremely low blood sugar that could cause her problems, if she was not careful. She eats regular meals that contain a lot of protein and stays away from sugar and caffeine. Margot uses relaxation therapy on a regular basis to keep the amount of cortisol and adrenaline from damaging her central nervous system. Stress and anxiety can set off a release of dangerous chemicals into the bloodstream. Margot's life turned around and her focus is positive.

Patients who experience dental anxiety and tension when they need extensive dental work have had excellent success using GABA prior to their appointments. Before I had a root canal I took two Anxiety Control capsules thirty minutes before my appointment and two more two hours later. I was able to relax during the procedure and felt much less tension since GABA prevented the release of unpleasant memories stored in the amygdala for playback at a later time. Dental visits for me are usually unpleasant, and GABA restores the neurotransmitters and slows down the anxiety-related messages. Patients who experience white-coat anxiety and fear before they visit their doctors have much less discomfort if they use GABA prior to their appointment. Muriel MacFarlane, R.N., M.A., in her book, *Panic Attacks, Anxiety, and Phobia Solutions Handbook,* describes her experience with GABA 750 for anxiety. She found opening the capsule and using it directly under her tongue was very effective, and quickly absorbed for relief. People with fear of flying use this same technique and report they have less anxiety during takeoffs and landings that seem to be the dreaded part of flying. I suggest using a combination of GABA and relaxation techniques. Deep breathing alone will elevate the serotonin level in the brain and reduce anxiety. Remember, a relaxed muscle cannot contract in spasms or respond to anxiety. When you combine GABA and magnesium, you address the two nutrients depleted first in stressful situations.

John is a 36-year-old attorney who had to drive on a busy expressway twice daily to and from work. When he came in to see me for chronic stress and anxiety he described his daily drives as feelings of intense fear and loss of control. He had recurrent nightmares about being closed in on the expressway and having an accident. John had never had an accident, but for a period of two years he rode with a friend. This caused him to experience a great deal of fear. His physician put him on Xanax, but his intense fear was still there. So he discontinued his Xanax, and realized he had a problem with his brain chemistry. To analyze his brain chemistry, we ran an amino acid analysis. The results disclosed a total neurotransmitter imbalance, and John was running on empty. His amygdala recorded his two years of intense fear while riding with someone else, and then began playback anytime John was under stress. I placed John on a balanced neurotransmitter complex and two Anxiety Control, twice daily with GABA 375 mg under his tongue, as needed. He also learned conditioned relaxation to use while he was driving. I instructed John to use the GABA 375 mg just before the expressway. He progressed, but still had anger and fearful dreams—this was his fear of loss of control and anger toward his friend who drove too fast. I encouraged him to face his friend and tell him the problems he had caused. John made the phone call, and a few weeks later he felt much more relaxed and in control. John had been a victim of someone else's anger while driving. If he had not addressed his problems, his anxiety and fear would have developed into a full-blown phobia, related to driving and the expressway.

A study conducted by Frederick Petty, M.D. at the Veterans Affairs Medical Center in Dallas, reflected GABA levels were significantly lower in males with primary unipolar depression disorders than in healthy subjects. The plasma GABA levels of depressed patients were 40% below those of the controls. The GABA levels correlated positively with the duration of their illness and negativity with the age of onset of the mood disorder. Dr. Petty established GABA levels might be a biochemical marker of vulnerability to depression, as opposed to being a consequence of the illness. Low GABA levels with depression supports the biogenic amine hypothesis of depression.

A report in the *American Journal of Obstetrics and Gynecology* states GABA tends to have lower than normal levels in seizure patients with epilepsy. Seizure prone preeclamptic patients (hypertensive condition during late pregnancy that can lead to seizures) also have decreased brain GABA concentrations. GABA is very effective in the brain chemistry of epileptics. A seizure occurs when the GABA system crashes. Each neuron affects only a limited number of cells. If the GABA level is deficient, the GABA system goes out of whack and tens of thousands of neurons send messages too fast, too many, and simultaneously, resulting in seizures. The key is to keep the brain message system in balance by keeping the GABA level in needed amounts.

Scientific evidence collected over the past 20 years demonstrates the theory that those who have a problem with addiction have a deficiency of GABA, serotonin, glutamine, and other neurotransmitters. Alcoholism is a genetic disorder with GABA, dopamine, and serotonin defects in the brain chemistry. These deficiencies can have a genetic marker and cause predispositions to alcoholism, and use of recreational or mind-altering prescription drugs. Proper supplementation of needed neurotransmitters and GABA corrects these deficiencies. A major pattern of addictive behavior includes constant drug cravings and feelings of loss of control. Chronic use of mind-altering drugs causes an imbalance in the brain chemistry. The three major factors that cause addiction are stress/anxiety, genetics, and chronic abuse.

Research done by Roger Williams at the Clayton Foundation at the University of Texas, disclosed that those who have alcoholic behaviors have a definite deficiency of glutamine. Glutamine converts to GABA in the brain. Dr. William's research pointed to the theory of "biochemical individuality." This theory details that no two people will have the same brain requirements for amino acids, vitamins, and minerals. Why then, do the drug companies subscribe to the theory that everyone with anxiety needs Xanax or Prozac? Prescribed addiction is one of the most pervasive problems in the world. Mood-altering drugs such as Zoloft, Prozac, Sarafem, Paxil, Serzone, Celexa, and Effexor (all are SSRIs) work by targeting specific chemical messengers or neurotransmitters in the brain. Neurotransmitters send thought commands from one nerve cell to another. The drugs suppress all feelings of happiness, fear, pain, grief, and depression. These drugs block excitatory messages as well as use the available serotonin, which affect moods and the perception of pain.

Fear, anxiety, panic, and depression are a complex syndrome resulting from the failure of specific neurotransmitters, the chemical language of the brain to go from one cell to the next. The nerve cell or neuron should fire smoothly across the synapse in the brain.

GABA Receptor Site

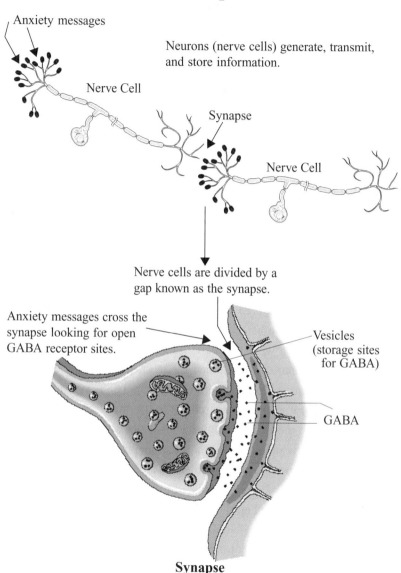

Neurons (nerve cells) generate, transmit, and store information.

Anxiety messages

Nerve Cell

Synapse

Nerve Cell

Nerve cells are divided by a gap known as the synapse.

Anxiety messages cross the synapse looking for open GABA receptor sites.

Vesicles (storage sites for GABA)

GABA

Synapse

Anxiety messages chemically cross the synaptic gap and reach receptors when GABA is not present or low. When GABA receptor sites are full, messages do not easily cross synapse and to the cortex causing increased anxiety.

Most addictive drugs change the effect of neurotransmitters on neurons in a negative way. Drugs can damage your intellectual property by blocking nerve impulses, preventing neurotransmitters from getting where they should be. Addictive drugs can also lower the production of needed neurotransmitters. Many antidepressants just slow down the reuptake of neurotransmitters into the brain synaptic terminals. This interferes with the recycling of neurotransmitters back into the cells that release them. Drugs may overstimulate the neurons inhibiting central nervous system function. The overstimulation disturbs the body's delicate mechanisms with toxic drugs; this is irrational, and leads almost invariably to increased anxiety, addiction, and despair.

The major focus of the drug companies is to create a line of drugs to focus on inhibitory neurotransmitters such as GABA. Eli Lilly, manufacturer of Prozac, is requesting approval from the FDA to use Prozac for children. The company already has on the market a peppermint-flavored version of Prozac. And where Prozac leads, all other manufacturers of antidepressants and tranquilizers will be sure to follow. The drug companies are looking for a new market in teen and children since the adult market has begun to look for alternatives to mind-altering drugs. The reason millions of dollars *are not* spent on research of GABA and other nutrients is money. You cannot patent a natural substance and make billions. With amino acids such as GABA, glutamine, tyrosine, and 5-HTP, the root of the problem can be addressed and corrected. Extensive research by psychopharmacologists in the last twenty years supports the theory that when the brain is given adequate amounts of amino acids, the building blocks for neurotransmitters, behavior is normal. If you have too little or inadequate amounts of amino acids, you may have constant anxiety, drug dependency, or a possibility of increased alcohol intake. A deficiency of GABA, the master controller, can lead to symptoms of restlessness, nervous stomach, increased muscle tension, and pain. The special combination pain formula of GABA, DL-phenylalanine, magnesium, ashwagandha, and boswellia prove effective in relieving stress or anxiety-induced pain. Amino acids such as GABA do not plug up brain chemicals; they restore them.

GABA acts as a muscle relaxant and its receptor sites are widely distributed throughout the brain, including regions normally associated with pain transmission and suppression. Pain messages are excitatory. GABA is inhibitory. GABA slows down and blocks the excitatory levels of brain cells that are about to receive pain-related incoming messages. Thus, when the cortex receives the message, it does not overwhelm you with pain or fear of pain. Both the head brain and the stomach brain have major receptor sites for pain messages; when the GABA receptors are empty, you can be overwhelmed with pain and anxiety-related messages. The pain, stress, anxiety cycle, then takes over.

Studies at major university pain clinics demonstrated that the brain produces many hormone-like chemicals with a close resemblance to morphine. These morphine-like chemicals are called endorphins because they are produced by the body and are 500 times more powerful than morphine. Endorphins regulate and control pain transmission. Endorphins are inhibitory neurotransmitters as is GABA in the brain and nervous system. The fear of pain begins a cycle of pain messages traveling from the amygdala in the limbic system to the cortex. A situation that caused you to experience pain, a headache, digestive problems, or anxiety, will reproduce those same symptoms when you are in a similar situation. Memories of unpleasant experiences are imprinted into the brain through the amygdala, the storehouse of all memories and emotions.

The preventative medicine measure: use proper amounts of nutrients such as GABA, glutamine, glycine, DLPA, and magnesium. Magnesium is the number one stress mineral. When your magnesium level is low, your pain is intensified, and muscles

Major Inhibitory Neurotransmitters Are Depleted by

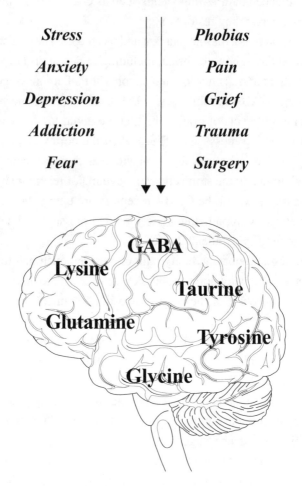

Receptors sites for major inhibitory neurotransmitters are found throughout the central nervous system (CNS), brain, and body. GABA cannot be stored. Stress, anxiety, depression, trauma, pain, and grief use available neurotransmitters. When the GABA switch is *on,* the brain is not flooded with adrenaline. GABA stores must be replaced on a regular basis by feeding the brain with neurotransmitters that come from amino acids and the cofactors, B6, and magnesium.

contract. The correct combination of amino acids in a balanced formula is extremely important. A shotgun approach is like band-aid first aid. Pain is a message, a message that something is wrong. Many times the problem is your own deficiency. Brain cells must have food in the form of amino acids. This creates the vital neurotransmitters that slow down the busy limbic system network. Pain will decrease as you address the nutritional needs of your brain and body. Remember, whatever the brain tells the body to do, the body will do!

The Pain & Stress Center followed twelve patients using the Pain Control formula containing GABA, DLPA, magnesium, boswellia, ashwagandha, and B6. The patients had been diagnosed with chronic pain and stress syndrome. After using the Pain Control formula morning and afternoon for six weeks, all reported a remarkable improvement and a decrease in pain. Patients presented with various symptoms of chronic stress with recurrent muscle spasms in the head, neck, and shoulders. Interviews with patients disclosed long-term problems with anxiety, depression, and grief. Patients were given a combination of Anxiety Control, Pain Control, and Mag Link plus 5-HTP at bedtime. Within the first week, half the patients reported less morning stiffness, headaches, and muscle spasms. Those patients, whose problems were more intense at night, added GABA, 750 mg, upon awakening. For best results, GABA 750 should be opened, mixed in water (such as 8 ounce glass) and taken as needed during the night. For those who suffer chronic anxiety, nighttime is especially difficult. At night the subconscious is extremely active, and unresolved anxiety floods the brain with anxiety and panic. Buried in your subconscious is the story of your life, and traumatic experiences are like old tapes that play over and over. *Thoughts you suppress* during the day surface at night in your sleep cycle, and remains in your subconscious as *unresolved* anxiety.

In *Lancet,* August 14, 1982, a research report about tranquilizers

and GABA transmission clearly stated that GABA is a major inhibitory neurotransmitter in the central nervous system. Amino
acids that raise the brain's GABA concentration possess a sedative,
anticonvulsant property. Research has established that GABA plays
an important role in epilepsy. This documentation was reported in
the text, *GABA Receptors in Mammalian Function,* by N.G. Bow-
ery, H. Bittinger, and H.R. Olpe. Data demonstrated pharmaco-
logical intervention at the GABA synapse lead to a reduction of
transmission-induced phenomena. The causative role of GABA is
supported by the fact that anticonvulsants facilitate transmission.

Dr. K. Berman at Mt. Sinai School of Medicine published an
extensive review in *Clinical Neuropharmacology* (1985) entitled
"Progabide: A New GABA Mimetric Electric Agent in type of
neurotransmitter deficiency. Dr. Berman sums up the research and
results of the chemistry, the role of GABA, and the influences in
the central nervous system. In 1985 the most valid research published on GABA related to anxiety. In 2001 GABA's benefits are
still being explored. GABA, not only aids anxiety sufferers, but
also lessens muscle tension, and aids Parkinson's symptoms, as
well as inhibits the desire for alcohol and cocaine. This extremely
versatile amino acid is making major contributions to aid those
suffering from pain, stress, anxiety, grief, and addiction.

Neurobiologists report about 30% of the brain's synapses, the
gap between the nerve cells, use GABA as their inhibitory neurotransmitter. When anxiety-related messages cross the synapse,
if the GABA receptors are empty, the messages then have a clear
path to the cortex in the limbic network. If the received messages
overwhelm the cortex, physical symptoms of anxiety and panic
will follow. Major symptoms include increased heart rate, increased
blood pressure, increased sweat gland activity, increased muscle
activity, and gastrointestinal instability. Such changes reflect a
major decrease of the inhibitory neurotransmitters, GABA, glycine, glutamine, and taurine. There are glycine receptors present

among the GABA receptors in the synapses. GABA, glycine, and taurine are the major inhibitory neurotransmitters in the brain and central nervous system (CNS). These neurotransmitters maintain a balance between the limbic system and the rest of the brain for orderly communication. In the best-selling book, *Inside the Brain,* Ronald Kotulak states glycine helps trigger brain cells to fire electric charges and speed learning. A brain cell fires an electric charge that rewires itself as a new memory is formed, so it can send the information to other cells.

Drugs...

- No drug currently in wide use—medical or recreational—addresses the root of neurotransmitter problems.

- Drugs merely stimulate temporary excessive release of preexisting neurotransmitter stores.

- Drugs do not increase the production of neurotransmitters.

- This fact explains why drugs often lose their effect over time with chronic use—once preexisting stores of neurotransmitters are exhausted, the drug is unable to stimulate the brain.

Be Aware . . .

If you are taking prescription drugs, *DO NOT JUST STOP TAKING THEM!*

Withdrawal reactions *can occur.*

Know the withdrawal symptoms, so if you experience some of them, you won't be surprised.

Consult your physician or a qualified health care professional for help.

5
GABA,
Anxiety and Panic Disorders

According to the National Institute of Mental Health (NIMH), some 25 million people will suffer from some form of anxiety disorder in their lifetime. Recent figures reported from NIMH show between 8 and 9 million people afflicted. However, these figures reflect only those who have sought help or treatment in some way. Millions suffer in silence, fearful of peer pressure.

One such individual was a 43-year-old R.N. named Jackie. Jackie was only semi dysfunctional because of her anxiety and panic attacks. Some days she felt like she could not cope with the constant feelings of tightness in her chest, racing heart, intermittent irregular heartbeats, churning stomach, and a fear of driving. Jackie had a complete physical and her physician found no physical problems. He suggested she talk to a psychiatrist who prescribed Xanax, just to take the edge off. What her psychiatrist did not tell her was even a few weeks of daily Xanax use can lead to dependency. Whatever Jackie's problem was, she did not need Xanax, or any of its chemical cousins, especially since she had a history of alcohol abuse. Jackie's father was an alcoholic and her mother had had problems with benzodiazepines (Valium). This predisposed Jackie to a possible addiction problem. After two weeks she tapered off the Xanax, and began to search for answers.

She understood brain chemistry and knew she must have some type of neurotransmitter deficiency. Jackie came to see me, and I ran an amino acid analysis. The results reflected she had a major deficiency in GABA, glycine, taurine, and tryptophan, as well as magnesium. Jackie began a nutritional support program using the needed nutrients to bring her brain chemistry into balance. The magnesium regulated her heartbeat so she no longer experienced premature beats (PVC's) and her heart rhythm was slow and steady. The amino acids created the neurotransmitters she desperately needed.

Through a series of counseling sessions, we were able to uncover some of her major problems. Jackie, because of her traumatic childhood, repressed her feelings rather than expressed them. She was carrying all of the anger, frustration, and fear from her childhood as well as her adult life. The other major problem was grief that she was finally able to release. She grieved for a love one lost from an accident a few years earlier. She did not know how to release the memories so she could heal. Anger is a very powerful emotion. When constantly repressed, it can cause major health problems. Combine this with unresolved grief, and you can become an emotional time bomb.

Jackie's GABA receptors were empty, and all of her anxiety-related messages went straight to her hippocampus where memories begin and are processed. The physical symptoms would follow, and she would lose control. Jackie never needed the Xanax or any other drug. She needed GABA and other neurotransmitters to restore her depleted brain.

A study in *Consumer Reports,* January 1993, told the whole story.

> "Xanax is just the latest in a long line of tranquilizers that have promised to deliver a psychiatrist's holy grail: relief from anxiety with no significant side effects. And like the pills that came before it, Xanax has fallen short!"

Consumer Reports issued a major indictment against not only Xanax, but Prozac and Halcion, both hot selling psychoactive drugs. They all have histories of extensive potentials for hazardous side effects and addiction.

Paul is a 43-year-old attorney whose job was filled with stress and anxiety. Over a period of two years, Paul found himself becoming so increasingly tense and anxious that he was having a difficult time in court. He suffered panic attacks daily and chronic insomnia at night. Paul found it so hard to concentrate and function that he went to his physician who prescribed Xanax, Zoloft, and Halcion. The medications were to little avail. He felt worse taking the drugs and stopped. He decided to take a brief leave of absence and get some help. He feared he would become housebound. Few days went by that he was not shaking and suffering heart palpitations.

A friend of Paul's gave him a copy of my book—*The Anxiety Epidemic*. The first book I wrote describing my own battle with anxiety, panic, and chronic pain. After reading the book Paul understood how GABA improves brain function and reduces anxiety. Paul came to see me, and I started him on a nutritional support program of Anxiety Control, Mag Link, B Complex, and Pain Control. His symptoms of anxiety began to diminish, and his heartbeat became more regular. He was able to drive again without fear and a stiff neck. Paul had allowed his stress to consume him, and his fear of failure became his major focus. He did not know how to relax or how to release his stress, so it took control of his life. His GABA receptors were empty, so all anxiety-related messages went directly into his limbic network. He used GABA 750 mg in water when he felt overwhelmed. The GABA did the trick—he was able to calm down. Paul has returned to work now and is much improved. He continues his nutritional supplement program and takes a few minutes each day to do deep-breathing exercises.

Deep breathing can change the chemistry of your brain and

slow down the overproduction of adrenaline. Thousands of patients like Paul suffer daily and turn to tranquilizers or antidepressants for relief. The relief becomes a dependency in the form of prescribed addiction. Drugs distort the brain chemistry and cause changes in perception and thinking. Drugs offer those who take them a passive approach to existence. *There is NO SUCH THING AS A TRANQUILIZER DEFICIENCY!*

According to Peter Breggin, M.D., author of *Toxic Psychiatry*, "The modern psychiatrist may have NO interest in *talking therapy.* Their training is devoted to medical diagnosis and physical treatment. Psychiatrists prescribe drugs. That is what they have been trained to do and if one drug doesn't work then they try another." If that does not work, they increase the dose.

In *Psychiatry at the Crossroads,* by John Paul Brody, M.D., and Keith H. Brodie, M.D., they summarize the concept of Psychiatry,

The Limbic System

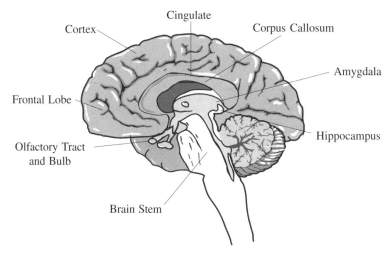

The limbic system includes the thalamus, hypothalamus, amygdala, parts of the reticular formation in the brain stem, and the limbic region of the central cortex. Limbic system functions deal mainly with behavior and emotions.

"We must hold firm in mind what psychiatry is, and what it is not. Psychiatry is not a science. It is a branch of medicine that cares for the subset of human misery that cannot be alleviated by the knife or a pill."

Over the past several years a new breed of healers has emerged—orthomolecular physicians and therapists. Although many are trained in the field of psychiatry they have expanded their education and training to include the use of amino acids, vitamins, and minerals. Caregivers such as these make a difference in a person's healing process and would not hesitate to use GABA and other amino acids rather than a toxic chemical to help a child or adult suffering from anxiety, depression, grief, or pain. With the help of GABA, thousands of people are free of chemical straight jackets and have conquered the fear within.

Dr. Candace Pert's research provides positive proof that GABA functions as the major inhibitory neurotransmitter in the brain, and the limbic network has the heaviest concentration of receptors. "And when we focus on emotions, it suddenly becomes very interesting that the part of the brain where peptides and receptors are the richest is also part of the brain ... implicated in the expressions of emotion." Dr. Pert's research with Michael Ruff disclosed neuropeptides and their receptors join the brain, glands, and immune system in a network of communication between brain and body—probably the biochemical substrate of emotion. Dr. Pert's book, *Molecules of Emotions*, gives an in-depth accounting of her years of research on brain function, as well as her body-mind theory.

All her theories support that the biological roots of anxiety, panic, fear, and grief are stored in the amygdala, master of the anatomy of memory. When a situation stimulates the amygdala in the limbic network, the firing of anxiety-related messages starts. The result of the firing depends on inhibition. GABA and its receptor sites, neurotransmitters and serotonin govern the inhibition. When your brain is depleted of GABA and other neurotransmitters, your body language and behavior reflect it. One of Dr. Pert's major breakthroughs is the explanation of why we have chronic pain. Repressed traumas caused by overwhelming emotion are stored in a body part—thereafter affecting our ability to feel that part of the body, or even, move it. The brain encodes experiences and messages for playback, especially when we are totally depleted of neurotransmitters and serotonin. We have a constant traffic of information that travels back and forth between the brain, the body, and the immune system. Neurotransmitters are very busy communicating with different cells in the body. With continued research such as Dr. Pert's, more uses for GABA will continue to emerge to help millions of anxious Americans.

In 1985 the TV series, *The Brain,* was shown on PBS; the documentary emphasized behavior as a product of brain function. Scientists gave a step-by-step description of what happens in the brain during prolonged stress, that begins the cycle of anxiety and panic.

Wrapped around the top of your brain stem deep inside your head is the limbic network. The limbic network makes up approximately one-fifth of the brain's space. Involved in this network is the amygdala, storehouse of memories, emotions, and especially, traumatic episodes. The hypothalamus is the size of a dime, yet its blood supply is one of the richest in the human body. From the hypothalamus come feelings of anger, rage, aggression, punishment, pleasure, sexual arousal, hunger, and thirst. The hypothalamus maintains the body's internal equilibrium due to its connections with the brain stem. When the hypothalamus is out of balance, problems such as compulsive eating or a total loss of interest in food can occur.

The locus ceruleus, located at the base of the brain, controls the brain's alarm hormone noradrenaline, or norepinephrine. When prolonged stress occurs, the locus ceruleus sends out surges of stress hormones that keep the body in a state of fight-or-flight. The first physical symptoms of an adrenaline overload are increased

Brain Feedback Loop

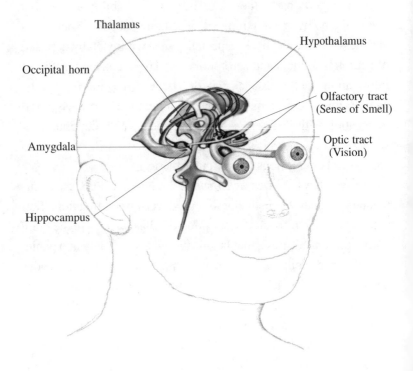

When you see, hear, or smell something that you associate with fear or anxiety, a signal flushes to the amygdala. The amygdala begins a continuous stimulation of the hippocampus where memories, both short-and long-term are stimulated. It constantly processes information relayed to the brain by the senses for comparison to previous experiences. The hippocampus receives and processes the signals for emotional responses such as anxiety, anger, rage, or intense fear. The thalamus is a relay station for the limbic system and passes the signals from sensory to motor nerves in the brain. Finally, the occipital horn and lobes receives messages where the feelings are translated into language and memory.

blood pressure, racing heart, and intense anger. Dr. Redfo iams of Duke University believes genetics or early childho velopment makes people more prone to hostility and anger. A genetic deficiency can cause a chronic deficiency of the neurotransmitter, serotonin. Anger, aggression, hostility, and loss of control are all symptoms of a low level of the master controller, serotonin.

The hippocampus is a tiny pea sized structure that sits just above the amygdala. The hippocampus has a major role in learning and memory, both short and long term. Unpleasant or painful memories are stored for playback during anxious episodes or events. Fear will usually be the result, and the physical symptoms follow.

Panic and anxiety attacks occur when the amygdala begins a nonstop firing of anxiety-related messages. Concurrently, physiological responses occur and the fight-or-flight syndrome comes into full bloom. For those who suffer from chronic stress syndrome and are totally depleted of GABA and other important nutrients, this means a dreaded loss of control. The constant bombardment of signals from the limbic network eventually overwhelms the cortex, and the abilities of the cortex and the rest of the limbic network go to pieces. This activity leads people to irrational fear and behavior. The ability of the cortex to communicate with the limbic network and the rest of the brain in an orderly manner depends critically on inhibition. GABA inhibits the cells from rapid firing, diminishing the excitatory level of the cell about to receive the incoming message. Continuous prolonged anxiety decreases GABA's ability to block messages, and finally anxiety messages literally bombard the cortex. A loss of control usually follows.

The brain is not a static organ. The cells constantly change with the influx of messages from the limbic network. Part of the amygdala's major function is to record negative experiences and play back what is frightening and could cause possible harm. The limbic system sorts the millions of thoughts that go through our minds, and sends them to the amygdala where they are encoded

Limbic System Bombarding the Cortex with Anxiety Messages

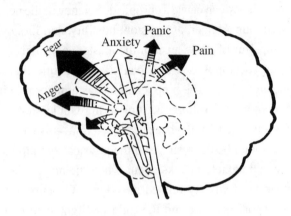

When bombarded with anxiety messages, the overwhelmed cortex
usually causes a loss of control.

for fear-based behavior. If a memory is encoded with extreme fear
into the amygdala, it causes almost uncontrollable memories that
trigger panic and intense fear. The amygdala, since it is closely
connected to the hypothalamus, controls the body's fight-or-flight
response. The key to control is to keep the stress hormones in
check to prevent the amygdala from overstimulation releasing fear
and anxiety. When the GABA switch is on, and the receptors are
full, we do not experience the constant dread or physical symptoms that follow a negative or fearful thought pattern. We become
aware of unpleasant situations, but not fearful, anxious, or uncom-
fortable.

Our emotions regulate what we perceive as reality and non-
reality. During a panic or anxiety attack when the brain is swim-
ming in adrenaline, we perceive everything to be real. This occurs
because your brain cannot filter out the sensory information of
what is real and what is not. Research at UCLA demonstrates how

memories are recorded. If the brain of an average 50-year-old could be emptied of all fear, anxiety, and memories, it had stored, and recorded on tape, the length of the tape would reach to the moon and back several times. When you stop and think about this, it makes you realize just how busy the brain is.

Neurotransmitters and neuropeptides govern the rate and amount of incoming messages. According to Candace Pert, Ph.D., in *Molecules of Emotion,* "Emotional experiences are much more likely to be recalled when we're in an upbeat mood, while negative emotional experiences are recalled more easily when we're in a down mood. Not only is memory affected by the mood we're in, but so is actual performance." Depression usually follows anxiety and a negative state of mind. Disturbances in the brain chemistry result from pervasive, constant fear or other profound emotional disturbances. Depression is more than just a mood. Depression creates a multitude of physical symptoms such as pain, headaches, intestinal problems, fatigue, appetite disturbances, and sleep problems.

Those who suffer from post-traumatic-stress disorder live in constant fear of when the next flashback or anxiety attack will occur. Their emotions, grief, and anger are all stored in their brain and body, and long after the danger passes, the fear persists in dreams. Flashbacks are not a new thought, but encoded memories. Many times the memories are fragmented; then again, they can be very precise replays of traumatic events that happened. Here again, the amygdala stores and releases them. GABA and other neurotransmitters have been very helpful to those who suffer from post-traumatic-stress disorder. Prescription drugs only block the memory and symptoms. A Balanced Neurotransmitter Complex + GABA nourishes the brain and protects it from stress.

The longer you allow fear to control your behavior, the more predisposed you become to a disease-oriented lifestyle. Your ability to handle stress and anxiety depends on your state of health.

Your state of health depends on your state of nutrition. Your state of nutrition depends on a well-planned program of amino acids, vitamins, and minerals to nourish your brain and body. Feed your brain, and let your healing begin!

The Brain

The brain . . .

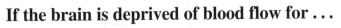

- Weighs 3 pounds.
- Uses 20% of the body's total energy output.
- Demands a constant supply of glucose and oxygen.
- Creates its own energy for the billions of neurons that must feed constantly.

If the brain is deprived of blood flow for . . .

- 15 to 20 seconds, unconsciousness results.
- 8 to 10 minutes and the brain begins to die.
- Brain cells do not reproduce as do other cells. Once the brain cells die, they are gone.

Rx for a healthy brain. . . Feed it!

- Your brain is controlled by your nutritional state.
- Your nutritional state is controlled by:
  - Nutrient intake.
  - Chronic stress.
  - Pain.
  - Disease.
  - Chemical Effects.

6
GABA and Sleep

GABA is very important for restful, anxiety-free sleep. During the sleep stage, thoughts suppressed during the day surface in nonstop dream form. Your dream state can be characterized by rapid transitions of daytime reality to nighttime emotionality and irrational behavior. In your dream state, you will do things that you would never think of doing in your awake stage. During sleep, you experience an increase in electrical activity. The increased activity of the limbic system and amygdala depletes GABA stores, thus, allowing an overpowering of dream images containing anxiety, fear, and even, depression.

Unresolved anxiety creates images in mysterious forms that cause you to awaken with alarm. GABA taken in water during the night slows down electrical activity and restores a balance in the brain. During sleep, serotonin, GABA, and other amino acids can deplete. GABA and 5-HTP should be taken before bedtime to allow you to have a peaceful night's sleep.

If you awaken and feel anxious, take GABA 375 mg in water; this restores your GABA level. Take several slow, deep breaths, and allow yourself to relax so you will go back to sleep. Remember deep breathing changes the chemistry of the brain and increases the master controller, serotonin. Studies suggest when your nervous system is under the influence of deep breathing and relaxation; it releases neurotransmitters including nitric oxide that potentiates GABA. As you continue to relax, you improve blood flow to all of your organs, and reduce levels of epinephrine and cortisol. You should feel the results within minutes.

The Chemistry of Anxiety and Stress

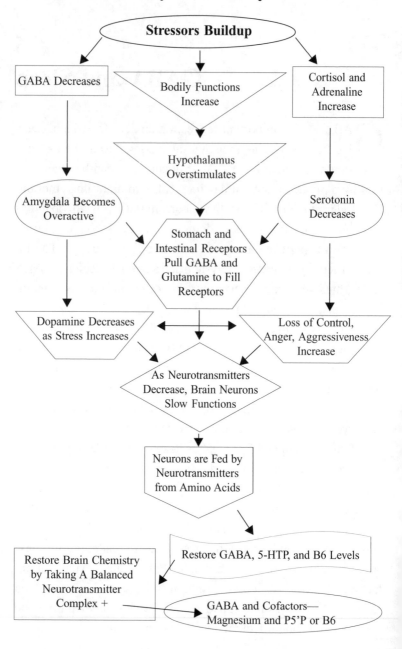

7
GABA and Memory

Recent research in the field of neuroscience allows us to see the brain function in action as it learns and remembers. This research opens a door that allows us to see in an understandable way what is going on inside our heads, even, during stressful and anxious events that cause memory failure. Two regions of the brain that show the highest levels of activity during an anxious period or traumatic episode, determine what you remember or forget. The temporal lobes, a part of the brain that, when damaged, can result in 75 to 80 % memory loss. The frontal lobes also have an impact on memory and how memory stores. Memory depends on how your brain encodes incoming thoughts or events.

If the GABA receptors are empty from prolonged anxiety, depression, or stress, thoughts and events encode as negative, unpleasant, or traumatic. When you recall that particular memory, your ability to remember details can be impaired. For example, a student studying for exams with an intense fear of failure, the fear impairs his ability to recall needed information. GABA controls the release of adrenaline and cortisol into the bloodstream. Your memory association is based on your brain chemistry. During stressful times your neurotransmitter production reduces; that in turn, reduces memory recall. If you fear you will forget words, visual images, or numbers, you set up an association with fear linking incoming information to the fear encoding

GABA, glutamine, and glycine stimulate memory and the production of neurotransmitters. The memory capacity of the human brain is effectively infinite depending on how the information is stored. Memory requires a certain degree of attention. A flood of neurotransmitters creates attention that turns important areas in the brain, on and off. Neurotransmitters hold the key to thought, memory, attention, and focus. A balanced neurotransmitter complex (BNC) supplies the brain with adequate neurotransmitters to improve mind, mood, memory, and behavior. BNC should be taken daily since the brain cannot store amino acids.

The doctor of the future
will give no medicine
but will interest his patients
in the care of the human frame,
in diet, and in the cause and
prevention of disease.

—Thomas A. Edison

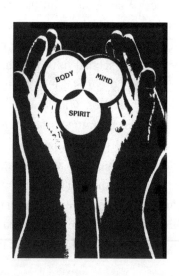

8
GABA Support Products

GABA 375 or 750 mg. GABA (Gamma Amino Butyric Acid) is a major inhibitory neurotransmitter. Stress and anxiety deplete GABA levels in the brain and body. GABA helps *cool* the brain. Amino acid deficiencies occur when we experience long periods of stress, anxiety, depression, or pain. The brain is then bombarded by anxiety signals that cause you to become anxious, tense, and out of control. GABA 750 has a natural calming effect. Dr. Julian Whitaker in *Health & Healing*, March 1994, described GABA 750. Recommended dosage is ½ capsule dissolved in water or under the tongue three times daily if your weigh less than 125 pounds. If you weigh over 125 pounds, dissolve one capsule in water or under your tongue three times daily. *Always use GABA, pharmaceutical grade, in capsule form.* Children should use GABA in a combination formula such as Brain Link or Anxiety Control.

Anxiety Control 24 (AC24) is a unique amino acid support formula. Anxiety Control combines amino acids, herbs, minerals, and essential cofactors to help relax the anxious or stressed mind and body. I spent several years researching and formulating the Anxiety Control formula. Anxiety Control was awarded a U.S. patent in October 1997. Anxiety Control contains the major inhibitory neurotransmitters in the brain: GABA, glycine, and glutamine. Neurotransmitters are the chemical language of the brain. B6 is the major cofactor for activation of amino acids in the body. The herbs, Passion Flower and Primula Officinalis, support an overstressed body and calm the central nervous system naturally. Anxiety Control 24 can be used all day or at night to feed the brain deficiencies created by today's stressful life-styles. AC24 can be used for teens and children who are anxious or overly active. Recommended dosage, *for anyone over 100 pounds,* is up to 4 capsules daily, in divided doses. Children weighing 50 to 100 pounds can take one capsule, twice to three times daily, divided.

B.N.C. + GABA. Neurotransmitters are the chemical language of the brain. B.N.C. + GABA provides your brain the needed nutrients to enhance maximum use of the brain. An unbalanced diet, anxiety and stress, plus other factors, can contribute to disturbances in amino acid metabolism. Many people have undetected impairments of their biochemistry that can either cause or complicate their health condition. Amino acids are intimately involved in metabolic regulation, and prove very useful as therapeutic agents that reverse the biochemical impairments related to amino acid metabolism. Amino acid therapy can be instrumental in correcting or reducing stress and anxiety, chronic fatigue, food and chemical intolerances, frequent headaches, recurrent infections, mental and emotional disturbances, hyperactivity, learning disabilities, neurological disorders, drug cravings, and eating disorders. B.N.C. + GABA mixes in fruit juice for rapid absorption. Recommended dosage is one teaspoon, two times daily.

Brain Link Complex is an amino acid complex that creates the neurotransmitter link for enhanced brain function. Brain Link is a total formula for daily use, and can be used in conjunction with all other supplements. Brain Link is the most complete neurotransmitter formula available on the market today. Brain Link is perfect for all ages, 1 to 100. Recommended dosage is by weight, children up to 75 pounds take two scoops; 75-120 pounds, take four scoops; and over 120 pounds, take six scoops daily in divided doses.

Mood Sync is a amino acid/herbal formula combining St. John's Wort, GABA, taurine, glutamine, 5-HTP, and B6. Mood Sync provides St. John's Wort, the depression herb, and 5-HTP to elevate the serotonin levels in the brain and body. GABA, glutamine, and taurine are inhibitory neurotransmitters that nourish the brain in times of stress, depression, anger, aggression, mood swings, and PMS. *NOTE: Do not take use if you are taking Selective Serotonin Reuptake Inhibitors (SSRIs) medications.*

Pain Control 24 is a special combination of amino acids and herbs that have special pain reducing properties. This combination has been used at the Pain & Stress Center in our pain program with excellent success. Pain Control is excellent for reducing stress-induced pain, but it is also a support formula for pain. Pain Control contains DLPA, Boswella, GABA, and Ashwagandha. For maintenance, use four capsules per day in divided doses, and up to six if needed. *NOTE: Do not take MAOs or tricyclic antidepressants with DL-phenylalanine (DLPA).*

Teen Link is a specialty formula for the active teen's or adult's brain. Teen Link is a complete neurotransmitter focus-support formula. It contains 5-HTP (5-Hydroxytryptophan), St. John's Wort, GABA, taurine, and glutamine, plus important cofactors to help

Symptoms of Serotonin Deficiencies

- Depression
- Anxiety/panic attacks
- Migraine headaches
- PMS
- Carbohydrate/sugar cravings
- Insomnia
- Obesity
- Fibromyalgia
- Alcoholism
- OCD (Obsessive Compulsive Disorder)
- Aggressive or violent tendencies
- Chronic Pain
- Hyperactivity

enhance the neurotransmitters in the brain. Teen Link helps support brain activity with smooth transmission signals between brain cells. 5-HTP and St. John's Wort help increase the serotonin levels in the brain. Serotonin is a key neurotransmitter in brain function. Serotonin is the neurotransmitter that enhances focus, elevates mood, reduces aggression, and helps reduce cravings for alcohol and carbohydrates. For maintenance, use one or two capsules morning and afternoon. *NOTE: Do not use if you are taking Selective Serotonin Reuptake Inhibitors (SSRIs) medications.*

5-HTP (5-Hydroxytryptophan) is the precursor to serotonin in the body. 5-HTP is about 10 times stronger than tryptophan, and is only one step biochemically away from serotonin. Serotonin is the master controller in the brain and body. The gastrointestinal tract has 80% of the receptor sites in the body while the brain has 1 to 2%. Serotonin produces a relaxed, calm, secure, mellow, uplifted, and tranquil mood. Serotonin helps with insomnia and pain. *NOTE: Do not use if you are taking Selective Serotonin Reuptake Inhibitors (SSRIs) medications.*

Tryptophan → 5-HTP → Serotonin (the Master Controller)

Liquid Serotonin is a special homeopathic 1X formula that contains serotonin in distilled water. Liquid Serotonin can be used by children or adults for acute anxiety, or to boost the serotonin levels in the brain and body to produce calm and tranquility. Homeopathic formulas work with the body by stimulating the body to produce more serotonin or other neurotransmitters.

GABA and Amino Acid Cofactors

B6 (Pyridoxine) or P5'P

Our bodies cannot function without enzymes, and every chemical reaction within the body starts with the enzyme triggers. Enzyme reactions start with B6 or P5'P (Pyridoxal 5' Phosphate), and serves as a catalyst so the body can digest amino acids (proteins), carbohydrates, and fats. B6 breaks down into P5'P, the biological form of B6. You should take B6 in a timed-release capsule (150 mg) that releases over 8 to 9 hours, or take P5'P. If you exceed 300 mg of B6 daily, you can develop irreversible neurotoxicity. Using P5'P instead of B6 protects against neurotoxicity, even in children.

Magnesium

Magnesium is an *essential* cofactor in over 300 enzyme reactions in the body, and plays an important role in the metabolism of GABA and other amino acids. Up to 70% of Americans are deficient in magnesium, and do not get enough from their diet. Magnesium is known as the stress mineral and is necessary for energy production and DNA replication, the basis of life.

Magnesium deficiency causes the release of more histamine that triggers an allergic reaction to a food, chemical, or environmental pollen. Ingestion of soft drinks, alcohol, and processed foods that are high in phosphates cause loss of magnesium. Medications such as asthma meds (theophylline), diuretics (lasix), being over 40 years of age, and diabetes increase the loss of magnesium from the body.

Supplement with magnesium chloride tablets such as Mag Link. Use 4 to 6 tablets, per day, divided throughout the day. If loose stools or diarrhea occur, decrease the dose by 1 tablet, or increase the interval between doses.

Alpha KG

Alpha KG and citric acid are part of the Krebs cycle, the chemical engine that generates energy for every cell. Alpha KG works with B6 and magnesium to metabolize GABA and amino acids for proper brain neurotransmitter production.

GABA-Mag Connection

Symptoms of
Magnesium *Deficiency*

- Anxiety
- Panic attacks
- Mitral valve prolapse
- Hypertension
- Chronic pain
- Back and neck pain
- Muscle spasms
- Migraines
- Fibromyalgia
- Constipation
- Fatigue
- Diabetes
- Hypoglycemia
- Spastic symptoms
- Chronic bronchitis, emphysema
- Vertigo (dizziness)
- Confusion
- Depression
- Psychosis
- Noise sensitivity
- Ringing in the ears
- Irritable Bowel Syndrome
- Cardiovascular disease
- Cardiac arrhythmias
- Atherosclerosis/Intermittent claudication
- Raynaud's disease (cold hands and feet)
- TIA's (Transient Ischemic Attacks-strokes)
- Asthma
- Seizures
- Kidney stones
- Premenstrual syndrome (PMS)
- Menstrual cramps
- Osteoporosis

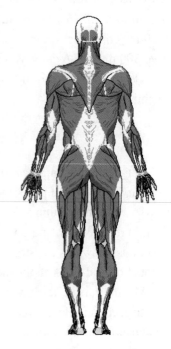

You have 657 muscles that need magnesium every second of every day. Magnesium is a cofactor for all amino acids.

For maximum benefit, add some magnesium in the form of magnesium chloride such as Mag Link. Try two tablets, twice to three times daily. If loose stools or diarrhea occur, decrease by one tablet or try increasing amount of time between doses. You should begin to feel a decrease in symptoms.

Warning: People with renal or kidney failure should not take magnesium without medical supervision.

For detailed information on magnesium deficiency symptoms, read *The Anxiety Epidemic* or *Heal with Amino Acids and Nutrients* by Dr. Sahley.

9
Product Information

There are many GABA formulas on the market, but not all contain the needed amounts of GABA. Your brain needs more than 100 mgs. of GABA to restore the level. *GABA in tablet form is not as effective as capsules.* The *purity* of amino acids and nutritional supplements is very important to your success. *Be selective.* Your body responds to what you absorb. Absorption is enhanced when you *use only pharmaceutical-grade and standardized herb products.* There are four grades of supplemental amino acids and nutritional products. They are in order of purity from least to purist: Food lot, Cosmetic, Pharmaceutical grade, and I.V. grade.

Pharmaceutical grade generally guarantees purity of product. Capsules are usually cleaner and purer than tablets, and *more bioavailable.* Tablets require fillers and binders plus the body has to break tabs down. When considering nutritional supplements, look for preservative-free and excipient-free products because they are better. Buy supplements free of preservatives, fillers, binders, or excipients of any kind. *Insist on pharmaceutical-grade products. Your body and brain will know the difference.*

For information on products and other books, call 1-800-669-225 or visit the Pain & Stress Center Website: http://www.painstresscenter.com

Physical Stress Reactions

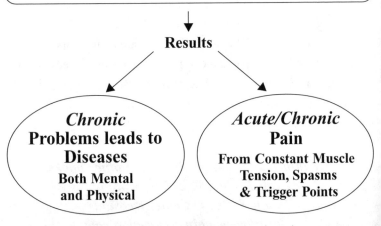

Within 24 to 48 hous after a stress-anxiety-anger reaction, major physical symptoms *can and do* occur.

Headaches	Diarrhea	Skin eruptions/acne
Face/Body pains	Constipation	Elevated blood pressure
Neck/Back pain	Pounding heart	
Trigger points	Increased sweating	Bladder Infections
Sleep loss	Increased anxiety	Ulcers
Upset stomach	Jaw clenching	

Results

Chronic **Problems leads to Diseases** **Both Mental and Physical**

Acute/Chronic **Pain** **From Constant Muscle Tension, Spasms & Trigger Points**

Physical stress reactions occur after major stress, anxiety, or anger.
Mental stress causes physical symptoms.

10
Xanax—
A Voyage into the Twilight Zone*

Xanax, America's hottest-selling tranquilizer, praised by some, condemned by many, has become one of the nation's most controversial drugs as a result of approval for use in the treatment of panic disorder, a severe form of anxiety. Panic disorder may be cured naturally without any hazard of adverse drug side effects. The condition is not life threatening, although it leaves its victims severely disabled. Often, the victim withdraws from most activities and lives in constant dread of the next panic attack.

Documents obtained from the Food and Drug Administration (FDA) under the Freedom of Information Act indicate no evidence exists that Xanax (a benzodiazepine tranquilizer produced by Upjohn) *cures* anxiety or panic disorder, nor that it is even *safe*.

The product does have FDA approval for *treating* both conditions. However, serious adverse effects were reported even in the short-term clinical trials (less than 10 weeks). The FDA required a clinical trial of Xanax (alprazolam) in order for Upjohn to obtain approval.

Xanax is a *therapy* with a great potential for harm. The drug does not effectively resolve the underlying biochemical basis of anxiety-state disorders. The *evidence* for the FDA approval was obtained from three very short-term studies. Several senior FDA officials expressed concern that there is no data to suggest that Xanax is safe over a long period or at higher dosages—yet, there are many patients who are being prescribed this drug for months, and even years!

Actually, there is compelling evidence that benzodiazepines, particularly Xanax, may be among the *more addictive* substances in the American drug marketplace. Thomas Temple, M.D., director of the FDA Office of Drug Evaluation, noted the potential for Xanax withdrawal phenomena was "clearly the area of main concern for two principal reasons. First, there is the matter of seizures. ... In addition, there is the issue of life long dependence, i.e., inability to discontinue therapy."

FDA Psychiatric Drug Products group leader, Thomas Laughren, M.D., agreed that much of Upjohn's information concerning withdrawal events was "often poorly organized and confusing." The official expressed "frustration that so little useful data have emerged... ."

Yet, the FDA has approved this drug in high dosages (up to 10 mg per day) for the treatment of panic disorder without evidence that it is safe for long-term prescription! At the highest dosage level (6 mg per day) administered in the short term studies subjects were having considerable difficulties with adverse side effects.

What do quotes from the new Xanax (Upjohn) product labeling reveal? "Demonstrations of the effectiveness of Xanax by systematic clinical study are *limited to four months duration* for anxiety disorder and *four to ten weeks* duration for panic disorder." Upjohn has aggressively marketed Xanax for a decade. Yet, no long-term studies exist on Xanax. Xanax sells for over $800,000 per kilo. What is their motive?

Upjohn admits, "Certain adverse clinical events, some life-threatening, are a direct consequence of *physical dependence* (addiction) to Xanax." These include a spectrum of withdrawal symptoms—the most important is seizures. Studies of patients with panic disorder show a high rate of rebound and withdrawal symptoms with Xanax. Other symptoms, such as anxiety and insomnia, were frequently seen during discontinuation.

The ability of patients to completely discontinue therapy with Xanax after long-term therapy has not been reliably determined. Withdrawal reactions may occur when dosage reduction occurs for any reason. "Withdrawal symptoms, including seizures, have been reported after only brief therapy with Xanax at doses within the recommended range for treatment of anxiety... Death has been reported in association with overdoses of alprazolam by itself."

Xanax has the potential to cause severe emotional and physical dependence in some patients, and these patients find it exceedingly difficult to terminate treatment. The following adverse events have been reported with the use of Xanax: seizures, hallucinations, depersonalization, taste alterations, diplopia, elevated bilirubin, elevated hepatic enzymes, and jaundice.

The necessary duration of treatment for panic disorder victims' responding to Xanax is unknown. A carefully supervised tapered discontinuation may be attempted, but evidence demonstrates that this is often difficult to accomplish without recurrence of symptoms and/or the manifestation of withdrawal phenomena.

The FDA has approved Xanax, a drug with unknown *long-term* consequences and potential for *addiction,* for a non-life-threatening condition that has been treated successfully by *non-drug* means! Xanax has become a major economic success story for the Upjohn Company—small wonder with its habituating potential and immediate appeal for sufferers of panic and anxiety disorders desperately seeking relief.

In the end, the long benzodiazepine tranquilizer voyage is a journey into the darkest side of the twilight zone—another world's timeless hell for those that are lured there seeking calm, and yet finding unrelenting heightened anxiety and abject misery.

*Excerpt from Xanax—A Voyage into the Twilight Zone by Max Ricketts. Read Max Ricketts' story of addiction in his book, *The Great Anxiety Escape.*

Bibliography

Aggleton, John P., ed. *The Amygdala*. New York, NY: Wiley-Liss, Inc., 1992.

Balch, James F. and Balch, Phyllis A. *Prescription for Nutritional Healing, A-to-Z Guide to Supplements*. Garden City Park, NY: Avery Publishing Group, 1998.

Bergmann, Kenneth J. "Prozabide: A New GABA-Mimetic Agent in Clinical Use." *Clinical Neuropharmacology*. Vol. 8, No. 1, 1985. New York: Raven Press, pp. 13–23.

Blakeslee, Sandra. "Complex and Hidden Brain in the Gut Makes Stomachaches and Butterflies." *New York Times*, January 23, 1996, pp. C1–3.

Bland, Jeffrey, ed. *Medical Applications of Clinical Nutrition*. New Canaan, CN: Keats Publishing, Inc., 1983.

Brady, John Paul and Brodie, H. Keith H. *Psychiatry at the Crossroads*. Philadelphia, PA: The Saunders Press, 1980.

Braestrup, Claus and Nielsen, Mogens. "Neurotransmitters and CNS Disease." *The Lancet*. November, 1982, pp. 1030–1034.

"The Brain" series. Public Broadcasting Service, January 1985.

Braverman, Eric R. and Pfeiffer, Carl C. *The Healing Nutrients Within*. New Canaan, CN: Keats Publishing, Inc., 1987.

Breggin, Peter R., M. D. *Toxic Psychiatry*. New York, NY: St. Martin's Press, 1991.

Breggin, Peter R., M. D. and Breggin, Ginger Ross. *Talking Back to Prozac*. New York: St. Martin's Press, 1994.

Carter, Rita. *Mapping the Mind*. Berkeley: University of California Press, 1998.

Challem, Jack Joseph. "Everything You Need to Know About Amino Acids." *Health Quarterly*. Winter, 1982. pp. 13, 60–61.

Chweh, A.Y., et al. "Effect of GABA Agonists on Neurotoxicity and Anticonvulsant Activity of Benzodiazepines." *Life Sciences*. Vol. 36, No. 8, 1985, pp. 737–744.

Colby-Morley, Elsa. "Neurotransmitters and Nutrition." *Journal of Orthomolecular Psychiatry*. First Quarter 1983, pp. 38–39.

Cooper, Jack R., et al. *The Biochemical Basis of Neuropharmacology. 5th Ed*. New York: Oxford Press, 1986.

Cowen, P.J. and Nutt, D.J. "Abstinence Symptoms After Withdrawal of Tranquilizing Drugs: Is There a Common Neurochemical Mechanism?" *The Lancet*. August 14, 1982, pp. 360–362.

Doheny, Kathleen. "Panic Attacks: A Debilitating Disorder for Millions." *Health Express*. June 1983, pp. 60–61.

Downs, Robert and Van Baak, Alice. "The Amazing Power of Amino Acids, Part I." *Bestways*. January 1982, pp. 74–75.

Downs, Robert and Van Baak, Alice. "The Amazing Power of Amino Acids, Part II." *Bestways*. February 1982, pp. 56–58.

Dunne, Lavon J. *Nutrition Almanac*. 3rd Ed. New York: McGraw-Hill Publishing Co., 1990.

"Emotions in Pain." *Current Concepts on Pain and Analgesia*. Vol. 5, No. 1, pp. 1–2.

Essman, W.B., ed. *Nutrients and Brain Function*. New York, NY: Karger, 1987.

Functional Assessment Resource Manual. Asheville, NC: Great Smokies Diagnostic Laboratory, 1999.

Gaby, Alan. *Magnesium*. New Canaan, CT: Keats Publishing, Inc., 1994.

Gelenberg, Alan J., et al. "Tyrosine For the Treatment of Depression." *American Journal of Psychiatry*. May 1980, pp. 622–623.

Gerson, Michael R. *The Second Brain*. New York: HarperCollins Publishers, 1998.

Gitlin, Michael J. *The Psychotherapist's Guide to Psychopharmacology*. New York, NY: The Free Press, 1990.

Grant, Larry A. "Amino Acids in Action." *Let's Live Magazine*. August 1983, pp. 61–64.

Guyton, Arthur C. *Basic Human Neurophysiology*. Third Edition. Philadelphia: W. B. Saunders Company, 1981, pp. 207–217, 223.

Hammond, Edward J. and Wilder, B. J. "Gamma-Vinyl GABA: A New Antiepileptic Drug." *Clinical Neuropharmacology*. Vol. 8, No. 1, 1985, pp. 1–12.

Hoffer, Abram and Walker, Morton. *Orthomolecular Nutrition*. New Canaan, CN: Keats Publishing, Inc., 1978.

Hoffer, Abram and Walker, Morton. *Putting It All Together: The New Orthomolecular Nutrition*. New Canaan, CN: Keats Publishing, Inc., 1996.

Iverson, Leslie L. "Neurotransmitters." *The Lancet*. October 23, 1982. pp. 914–918.

Kaplan, Harold I, Freedman, Alfred, and Sadock, Benjamin. *Comprehensive Textbook of Psychiatry*. Vol. 3. Baltimore: Williams and Wilkins, 1980.

Kolata, Gina. "Your Hungry Brain." *American Health*. May/June 1983, pp. 45–50.

Kotulak, Ronald. *Inside the Brain*. Kansas City, MO: Andrews and McMeel, 1996.

Lee, William H. "Amazing Amino Acids." New Canaan, CN: Pine Grove Pamphlet Division of Keats Publishing, Inc., 1984.

Leonard, B.E. *Fundamentals of Psychopharmacology.* New York, NY: John Wiley & Sons, 1992.

Lesser, Michael. *Nutrition and Vitamin Therapy.* New York: Bantam Books, 1981.

Locke, Steven M.D. and Colligan, Douglas. *The Healer Within.* New York, NY: Signet, 1987.

MacFarlane, Muriel K. *Panic Attacks, Anxiety and Phobia Solutions.* Encinitas, CA: United Research Publications, 1996, pp. 254–256.

Moyers, Bill. *Healing and the Mind.* New York, NY: Main Street Books, Doubleday, 1993.

"Overcoming Nutritional Deficiencies Behind Anxiety, Attention Deficit and Hyperactivity Disorders." *Health/Science Newsletter.* June, 1996. pp. 1–8.

Pearson, Durk and Shaw, Sandy. *Life Extension.* New York: Warner Books, Inc., 1982.

Pert, Candace B. *Molecules of Emotion.* New York, NY: Scribner, 1997.

Pfeiffer, Carl C. *Nutrition and Mental Illness: An Orthomolecular Approach to Balancing Body Chemistry.* Rochester, VT: Healing Arts Press, 1987.

Pinchot, Roy B, ed. *The Brain, Mystery of Matter and Mind.* New York: Torstar Books, 1984.

Pines, Maya. "What You Eat Affects Your Brain." *Readers Digest.* September 1983, pp. 54–58.

Restak, Richard M. *Receptors.* New York, NY: Bantam Books, 1994.

Restak, Richard. *The Brain.* New York: Bantam Books, 1984.

Ricketts, Max with Bien, Edwin. *The Great Anxiety Escape.* La Mesa, CA: Matulungin Publishing, 1990.

Rogers, Sherry A., M.D. *Pain Free in 6 Weeks.* Sarasota, FL: Sand Key Company, Inc., 2001.

Rogers, Sherry A., M.D. *Tired or Toxic?* Syracuse: Prestige Publishing, 1990.

Rogers, Sherry A., M.D. *Wellness Against All Odds.* Syracuse, NY: Prestige Publishing, 1994.

Roland, Per E. *Brain Activation.* New York, NY: Wiley-Liss, 1992.

Sahley, Billie J. and Birkner, Katherine M. *Breaking Your Prescribed Addiction.* San Antonio, TX: Pain & Stress Publications®, 1998.

Sahley, Billie J. and Birkner, Katherine M. *Heal with Amino Acids and Nutrients.* San Antonio, TX: Pain & Stress Publications®, 2000.

Shabert, Judy and Ehrlich, Nancy. *The Ultimate Nutrient Glutamine.* Garden City Park, NY: Avery Publishing Group, 1994.

Schatzberg, Alan F., M. D. and Nemeroff, Charles B., M.D., Ph.D. *Textbook of Psychopharmacology.* Washington, DC: American Psychiatric Press, Inc., 1995.

Slagle, Priscilla. *The Way Up From Down.* New York: St. Martin's Press, 1992.

Smith, Bernard H. and Rosich-Pla, Antonio. "The Biochemistry of Mental Illness." *Psychosomatics.* April 1979, pp. 278–283.

Society of Neuroscience. Washington, D.C., 1999.

Whitaker, Julian. *Dr. Whitaker's Guide to Natural Healing.* Rocklin, CA: Prima Publishing, 1995.

Whitaker, Julian. *Health & Healing.* March, 1994. Vol. 4. No. 3, pp. 1–4.

Whitcomb, Harold and Bronson, Phyllis. "Managing Women's Hormones Naturally." *Alternative Medicine Digest.* Issue 20, pp. 118–121.

Williams, Roger J. *Biochemical Individuality.* Austin, TX: University of Texas Press, 1979.

Williams, Roger J. and Kalita, Dwight K., eds. *A Physicians's Handbook on Orthomolecular Medicine*. New Canaan, CN: Keats Publishing, Inc., 1977.

Zucker, Martin. "Orthomolecular Psychiatry Update." *Let's Live Magazine*. November, 1982, pp. 31–32.

Glossary

Acetylcholine – is the major neurotransmitter at the junction between most nerves and muscles; acetylcholine also orginates in subcortical structures above the brain stem.

Amino acids – are the building blocks of proteins in the body. Amino acids are organic molecules that join to form different proteins.

Amygdala – is the storehouse of all emotions in the body. The amygdala is a pecan-shaped bundle of nerves that sits at the front of the limbic system in the brain.

Anticipatory Anxiety – leads to avoidance of situations or places in which stimulus might be present.

Bipolar disorder – is a mood swing disorder characterized by episodes of both depression and mania intermixed with periods of normal mood.

Blood Brain Barrier – is a protective barrier that prevents certain toxic chemicals and other substances in the bloodstream from entering the brain.

Brain stem – regulates vital body body functions including respirations, and heartbeat.

Central Nervous System (CNS) – contains the brain and spinal cord.

Cortisol – is a hormone produced by the adrenal cortex. Cortisol plays a role in the metabolism of glucose, proteins, and fats. During stress, cortisol levels increase in the body, and cause more utilization of neurotransmitters.

Cortisone – is a hormone in the body that converts to cortisol. Cortisone is a drug that is used as an anti-inflammatory, immunosuppressant, and for adrenal hormone replacement therapy.

Dopamine – is a neurotransmitter found in high concentrations in the basal ganglia region of the brain.

Empathy – is identification with and understanding another person's situation, emotions, or motives.

Endorphins – are the neuropeptides that bind to opiate receptors in different areas of the brain to produce a potent analgesic effect. Endorphins are nature's morphine that is normally produced in the brain. *Endorphins* are inhibitory neurotransmitters that slow down the transmission of information in the brain and nervous system.

Enzymes – are proteins produced by cells that speed up biochemical reactions.

Frontal Cortex – records how and when a memory was acquired and the circumstances involved.

Generalized Anxiety Disorder – manifests as often, but not constant anxious feelings.

Genetic Predisposition – is a genetic vulnerability to a specific illness or disease that tends to run in families.

Hippocampus – is a U-shaped formation in the limbic system that plays an important role in learning, memory, and emotions.

Hyperventilation – is a symptom complex characterized by breathlessness, sighing, palpitation, sweating, tremor, aching of the chest, marked fatigue, and dizziness brought on by anxiety, fear, and panic.

Hypothalamus – is a small neuron cluster at the base of the forebrain, and is essential in coordinating the central nervous system.

Limbic system – lies at the base of the forebrain, and is involved with all emotions. The limbic system makes up one-fifth of the brain area.

MAOI or Monoamine Oxidase Inhibitor – is a type of antidepressant medication that works by blocking the action of the enzyme monoamine oxidase.

Medulla Oblongata – is located at the base of the brain that influences blood pressure, respirations, and swallowing.

Mood Swing Disorder – is commonly called "bipolar disorder." Usually Mood Swing Disorder represents a neurotransmitter deficiency.

Neurohormones – are hormones produced by glands within the brain such as pituitary or pineal gland.

Neuron – is a nerve cell. Neurons receive and transmit information from the outside and sends signals throughout the brain. Each neuron in the brain represents a small part of stored memory.

Neurotransmitters – are the chemical language of the brain. Neurotransmitters control behavior by reacting on specific receptors in the brain such as GABA.

Neuropeptides – influence information transfer within the brain.

Nitric Oxide – improves blood flow to the organs of the body and reduces the levels of epinephrine and cortisol.

Noradrenaline (Norepinephrine) – is the neurotransmitter and alarm hormone in the brain and body. Noradrenaline is a particular hormone needed to control problems of anxiety and depression. During the fight-or-flight response, this adrenaline-like compound releases.

Obsession – is a persistent compulsive preoccupation with an unwelcome idea, emotion, feeling, or impulse that forces itself into a person's consciousness and cannot be removed by reasoning.

Obsessive ideas – are thoughts that repetitively intrude into the consciousness and intrude into consciousness and interfere with the normal train of thought.

Obsessive-Compulsive Disorder (OCD) is a psychiatric disorder characterized by obsessive thoughts and compulsive behavior. OCD patients can also experience anxiety and panic attacks.

Orthomolecular – is the proper molecule in the brain. Linus Pauling coined the term.

Panic Disorder – is acute attacks of anxiety that causes a loss of control or fear of death. Panic disorder is a chronic illness characterized by recurrent acute anxiety attacks that have a definite onset and spontaneous termination.

Paresthesia – is a disorder of the skin, as prickling, burning, or numbness.

Phobias – are an intense fear of a particular situation, object, or place.

Post Traumatic Stress Disorder (PTSD) – refers to a set of specific types of reactions to a very stressful event, episode, or crisis.

Protein – is a molecule present in every cell and derives from amino acids.

Receptors – are specialized cells located in sense organs, skin, muscles, joints, brain, and throughout the body.

SSRI – is a *Selective Serotonin Reuptake Inhibitor*, a class of anti-depressant medications that prevents the reuptake of serotonin in the synapse or nerve cell. Some of the SSRIs include Prozac, Effexor, Effexor XR, Zoloft, Serzone, Paxil, Luvox, Celexa, and Sarafin.

Serotonin – is an inhibitory neurotransmitter, and is the brain's master impulse modulator for all emotions and impulses.

Situational Anxiety manifests as over anxious feelings regarding a particular situation or place.

Social Phobia – refers to intense anxiety regarding any social situation.

Synapse – is a gap between nerve cells (axon of one cell and dendrite of another) that carries neurotransmitters and nerve impulses between nerve cells.

Temporal Lobe – is the lobe of the cerebrum located laterally and below the frontal and occipital lobes. The temporal lobe contains nerve centers involving mood, memory, speech, hearing, smelling, vision, and learning.

Thalamus – is a relay center for sensory and motor information to and from the brain.

Tricyclic antidepressants – are a classification of antidepressant medications. Amitriptyline (Elavil), Imipramine (Tofranil), Desipramine (Norpramin), Nortriptyline (Aventyl or Pamelor), Protriptyline (Vivactil), and Doxepin are some of the most common. *Tricyclics should not be combined with tyrosine or phenylalanine.*

Suggested Reading

The Anxiety Epidemic by Billie J. Sahley, Ph.D.

> *The Anxiety Epidemic* is my own story of anxiety, fear, and panic from depression and grief—spanning the ten years of my life of suffering and my complete recovery *without* ever using prescription drugs.

Heal with Amino Acids and Nutrients by Billie J. Sahley, Ph.D. and Katherine M. Birkner, C.R.N.A., Ph.D.

Breaking Your Prescribed Addiction by Billie J. Sahley, Ph.D. and Katherine M. Birkner, C.R.N.A., Ph.D.

Awakening Intuition by Mona Lisa Schultz, M.D., Ph.D.

Breaking the Grip of Dangerous Emotions by Janet Maccaro, Ph.D., C.N.C

Depression Cured at Last by Sherry Rogers, M.D.

Inside the Brain by Ronald Kotulak

Pain Free in 6 Weeks by Sherry Rogers, M.D.

Magnesium by Alan R. Gaby, M.D.

Molecules of Emotion by Candace Pert, Ph.D.

Nutrition & Mental Illness by Carl C. Pfeiffer, M.D.

How to Heal Anxiety and Panic Disorder by Jan Wolterman
> (To Order this book, call 513-741-2055)

The Great Anxiety Escape by Max Ricketts

The Second Brain by Michael D. Gershon, M.D.

The Ultimate Nutrient, Glutamine by Judy Shabert, M.D., R.D., and Nanc Ehrich

Tired or Toxic by Sherry Rogers, M.D.

Toxic Psychiatry by Peter Breggin, M.D.

Your Drugs May Be the Problem by Peter Breggin, M.D.

5HTP, The Natural Serotonin Solution by Robert A. Passwater, Ph.D.

Index

Other Publications by Dr. Billie J. Sahley
Call 1-800-669-2256 to Order

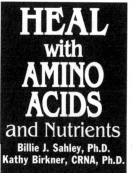

HEAL with AMINO ACIDS and Nutrients
Billie J. Sahley, Ph.D.
Kathy Birkner, CRNA, Ph.D.

- The brain is the most *poorly nourished* organ in the body.
- Amino acids create neurotransmitters, the chemical language of the brain, and are necessary for proper brain and body function.
- Learn how amino acids, control mind, mood, memory, and behavior.
- Learn how deficiencies of amino acids cause anxiety, panic, hyperactivity, pain, depression, more.
- Nutritional programs for stress, depression, grief, pain, headaches, insomnia, and others.
- A complete guide to all the amino acids.

Heal with Amino Acids **$12.95**

Addiction in America—Prescription Medications

- Finally, a step-by-step guide for withdrawal and maintenance from prescription meds or addictive substances.

- Withdrawal schedules and amino acid and nutrient replacement programs included.

- Learn what amino acids and nutrients to use to withdraw safely.

- Answers for your questions regarding medications, natural replacements, and a proven natural approach to recovery.

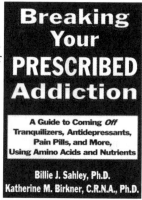

Breaking Your PRESCRIBED Addiction

A Guide to Coming *Off* Tranquilizers, Antidepressants, Pain Pills, and More, Using Amino Acids and Nutrients

Billie J. Sahley, Ph.D.
Katherine M. Birkner, C.R.N.A., Ph.D.

Breaking Your Prescribed Addiction **$9.95**

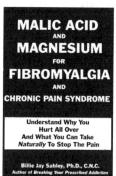

MALIC ACID AND MAGNESIUM FOR FIBROMYALGIA AND CHRONIC PAIN SYNDROME

Understand Why You Hurt All Over And What You Can Take *Naturally* To Stop The Pain

Billie Jay Sahley, Ph.D., C.N.C.
Author of *Breaking Your Prescribed Addiction*

Over 16 million Americans suffer from Fibromyalgia. This book explores what Fibromyalgia (FM) is and why you have it. Most importantly, it tells you how to get relief from the chronic pain, depression, and feelings of hopelessness.

A complete *easy-to-follow* program is outlined. Now you can begin to live again without pain. The nutritional approach offers hope and relief *without the side effects* experienced with medications.

This book gives you *answers* to help your healing process begin, and your constant pain diminishes. There is *natural help for FM.*

Malic Acid and Magnesium for Fibromyalgia **$3.95**

THE ANXIETY EPIDEMIC

A Wounded Healer Tells You How to Use GABA and Other Amino Acids to Control Anxiety and Panic

Billie J. Sahley, Ph.D.

There is No Such Thing as a Tranquilizer Deficiency!

A wounded healer takes you through her own five year battle with panic, fear, and phobias. Her healing came not from drugs, but vital nutrients that the brain must have to stop the dreaded fear.

Walk the path with this wounded healer and learn how to let your own healing begin.

If you suffer from anxiety, you *must* read this book.

Best book available on natural control of anxiety!

The Anxiety Epidemic $9.95

There are millions of children in this country who suffer from ADD or ADHD.

The orthomolecular program described in this book has been successfully used at the Pain & Stress Center to help hundreds of children whose symptoms range from mild to severe. This program corrects the brain deficiencies and imbalances WITHOUT DRUGS AND WITHOUT SIDE EFFECTS!

A complete guide for parents to follow that outlines a total orthomolecular approach for their children. A complete orthomolecular (drug-free) approach for parents to follow for positive, long-lasting results!

Control Hyperactivity A.D.D. Naturally $9.95

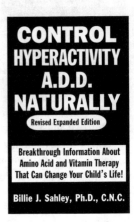

CONTROL HYPERACTIVITY A.D.D. NATURALLY

Revised Expanded Edition

Breakthrough Information About Amino Acid and Vitamin Therapy That Can Change Your Child's Life!

Billie J. Sahley, Ph.D., C.N.C.

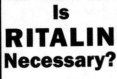

Is RITALIN Necessary?

THE RITALIN REPORT

Ritalin and Other Drugs Are NOT The Answer to ADD & ADHD—Amino Acids Offer *Safe, Effective Natural* Alternatives

Billie J. Sahley, Ph.D.

ADD has become #1 childhood and adult disorder!

Prescriptions for Ritalin have increased two and one-half fold in the last five years. If the trend continues, by the year 2000 over 20 million children will be on Ritalin.

Learn about Ritalin and other drugs that are currently being used to treat ADD.

This booklet is a must for parents, educators and health care practitioners. It details information not only about Ritalin, but other addictive medications used for children.

Is Ritalin Necessary? $5

Dr. Billie Sahley's Audio Tapes

Control of Anxiety

Anxiety/Panic Attacks

Stop Phobias

Anger

Fear

Control Stress with Amino Acids

Letting Go

Depression

Forgiving and Healing

Understand Who You Are

Fear of Sharing

Escape (Total Mind and Body Relaxation)

Each tape is $9.95 + P&H

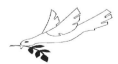

Panic is nothing more than a superficial
electrical charge at the nerve endings.

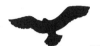

You can't live through tomorrow,
tonight let it go!

About the Author

Billie J. Sahley, Ph.D., is Executive Director of the Pain & Stress Center in San Antonio, Texas. She is a Board Certified Medical Psychotherapist-Behavior Therapist, Psychodiagnostician, and an Orthomolecular Therapist. She is a Diplomate in the American Academy of Pain Management. Dr. Sahley is a graduate of the University of Texas, Clayton University School of Behavioral Medicine, and U.C.L.A. School of Integral Medicine. Additionally, she has studied advanced nutritional biochemistry through Jeffrey Bland, Ph.D., Director of HealthComm. She is a member of the Huxley Foundation/Academy of Orthomolecular Medicine, Academy of Psychosomatic Medicine, North American Nutrition and Preventive Medicine Association. In addition, she holds memberships in the Sports Medicine Foundation, American Association of Hypnotherapists, and American Mental Health Counselors Association. She also sits on the Scientific and Medical Advisory Board for Inter-Cal Corporation.

Dr. Sahley wrote: *The Anxiety Epidemic*; *Control Hyperactivity/A.D.D. Naturally; Malic Acid and Magnesium For Fibromyalgia and Chronic Pain Syndrome; The Melatonin Report; Is Ritalin Necessary? The Ritalin Report;* and has recorded numerous audio cassette tapes. She coauthored *Breaking Your Prescribed Addiction,* and *Heal With Amino Acids and Nutrients*.

In addition, Dr. Sahley holds three U.S. patents for: SAF, Calms Kids (SAF For Kids), and Anxiety Control 24.

A Special Note . . .

While writing the second edition of this book we were faced with the loss of our beloved little boy named Scooter. Scooter was a little poodle that had been our constant love and companion for seventeen and a half years. On November 2, 1997, we were confronted with letting him go to Scooter heaven. We knew the grief and emptiness that would follow would leave a hole in our hearts for a long time to come. If we had not had the Anxiety Control to restore our GABA level, we're not sure how we would have made it through each long and lonely day. The loss of a pet who has been part of your family brings forth the same deep grief you feel when you lose a loved one.

I thank God daily for giving me the strength and courage to continue my research for natural substances such as GABA to help those who suffer grief, anxiety, depression, and pain.

Rest in peace my little Scooter! You're an angel in heaven now.

Dominus vobiscum

Dr. Billie Jay Sahley